T0334582

Noonan Syndrome

Noonan Syndrome

Characteristics and Interventions

Edited by

Amrit Bhangoo

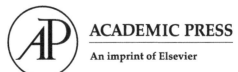

ACADEMIC PRESS

An imprint of Elsevier

Academic Press is an imprint of Elsevier
125 London Wall, London EC2Y 5AS, United Kingdom
525 B Street, Suite 1650, San Diego, CA 92101, United States
50 Hampshire Street, 5th Floor, Cambridge, MA 02139, United States
The Boulevard, Langford Lane, Kidlington, Oxford OX5 1GB, United Kingdom

Notices

Knowledge and best practice in this field are constantly changing. As new research and experience
broaden our understanding, changes in research methods, professional practices, or medical treatment
may become necessary.

Practitioners and researchers must always rely on their own experience and knowledge in evaluating
and using any information, methods, compounds, or experiments described herein. In using such
information or methods they should be mindful of their own safety and the safety of others,
including parties for whom they have a professional responsibility.

To the fullest extent of the law, neither the Publisher nor the authors, contributors, or editors,
assume any liability for any injury and/or damage to persons or property as a matter of products
liability, negligence or otherwise, or from any use or operation of any methods, products,
instructions, or ideas contained in the material herein.

Library of Congress Cataloging-in-Publication Data
A catalog record for this book is available from the Library of Congress

British Library Cataloguing-in-Publication Data
A catalogue record for this book is available from the British Library

ISBN 978-0-12-815348-2

For information on all Academic Press publications
visit our website at https://www.elsevier.com/books-and-journals

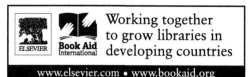

Working together
to grow libraries in
developing countries

www.elsevier.com • www.bookaid.org

Publisher: Stacy Masucci
Acquisition Editor: Tari K. Broderick
Editorial Project Manager: Megan Ashdown
Production Project Manager: Sreejith Viswanathan
Cover Designer: Vicky Pearson

Typeset by SPi Global, India

CONTENTS

CONTRIBUTORS

Robert P. Anthonappa
Paediatric Dentistry, Division of Oral Developmental and Behavioural Sciences, Discipline Lead and Program Convenor, UWA Dental School, The University of Western Australia, Nedlands, WA, Australia

Ashish Chogle
Division of Pediatric Gastroenterology, Children's Hospital of Orange County, Orange, CA, United States

Alicia Diaz-Thomas
Department of Pediatrics, University of Tennessee Health Science Center; LeBonheur Children's Hospital, Memphis, TN, United States

Francisco J. Garcia
Cypress Regional Hospital, Swift Current, SK, Canada

Moran Gotesman
Clinical Assistant Professor of Pediatrics, David Geffen School of Medicine at UCLA Pediatric Hematology/Oncology, Harbor-UCLA Medical Center, Torrance, CA, United States

Rishi Gupta
Division of Pediatric Gastroenterology, University of Maryland Medical Center, Baltimore, MD, United States

Alexander A.L. Jorge
Division of Endocrinology-Genetics (LIM/25), Discipline of Endocrinology, Faculty of Medicine, University of Sao Paulo (USP), Sao Paulo, Brazil

Nigel M. King
Faculty of Health and Medical Sciences, UWA Dental School, The University of Western Australia, Nedlands, WA, Australia

Alexsandra C. Malaquias
Division of Pediatric Endocrinology, Department of Pediatrics, Faculty of Medical Sciences, Santa Casa de Sao Paulo, Sao Paulo, Brazil

Ronak J. Naik
Division of Cardiology, Department of Pediatrics, Le Bonheur Children's Hospital, University of Tennessee Health Science Center, Memphis, TN, United States

Shalini Shah
Department of Anesthesiology & Division of Pain Management, University of California, Irvine, Orange, CA, United States

Sunil K. Sinha
Department of Endocrinology and Diabetes, Nationwide Children's Hospital, Columbus, OH, United States

Amit Soni
CHOC Children's Clinic, Orange; University of California-Irvine, Irvine, CA, United States

Minodora O. Totoiu
Division of Pediatric Neurology, Children's Hospital Orange County, University of California Irvine Medical Center, Orange, CA, United States

Peter Zhan Tao Wang
Western University, London, ON, Canada

Elias Wehbi
University of California, Irvine, CA, United States

Neda Zadeh
Genetics Center; CHOC Children's Hospital, Orange, CA, United States

AUTHOR BIOGRAPHY

Dr. Bhangoo is a pediatric endocrinologist with nearly a decade of experience teaching medical students, pediatric residents, pediatric endocrinology, and adult endocrinology fellows. Amrit P.S. Bhangoo, MD, is board certified in General Pediatrics and in Pediatric Endocrinology. He is currently serving as the Director of Research at CHOC Children's Endocrinology Division. He is also an attending physician at CHOC Children's and Assistant Professor of Pediatrics, University of California Irvine. Dr. Bhangoo earned his medical degree from India. In the United States, he underwent fellowship and residency training at Maimonides Children's Hospital of Brooklyn, New York. Before moving to California, he worked as an attending physician at SUNY Downstate Medical Center, New York. He has served as a senior editor of *Endocrinology, Diabetes & Metabolism Case Reports* and has served on editorial boards of *Journal of Pediatric Endocrinology* and *Endocrinology* and *Metabolic Research*. He has also served as a reviewer on multiple journals including *Pediatrics*, *Clinical Endocrinology*, *Journal of Clinical Endocrinology & Metabolism*, *Endocrine*, and the *European Journal of Endocrinology*. He has contributed book chapters to the *Textbook of Pediatric Endocrinology* (Taylor & Francis), *Pediatric Adrenal Diseases* (Karger), and *Genetic Steroid Disorders* (Elsevier) and has 35 peer-reviewed publications. He has invited authors from pediatric endocrinology, pediatric cardiology, genetics, pediatric urology, anesthesiology, pediatric hematology, pediatric gastroenterology, and dentistry to summarize the latest literature on Noonan syndrome and to compile it in one essential reference.

FOREWORD

Noonan syndrome is a relatively common multiple congenital abnormality syndrome and presents with a wide range of defects with serious life-threatening congenital heart defects to short stature, cryptorchidism, feeding difficulties, delayed language development, and poor long-term educational achievements on the mild end of the spectrum. The incidence of Noonan is described between 1:1000 and 1:2500 which is more prevalent than Turner syndrome, which is much more well-understood condition [1–3]. This current book was written to compile various reviews, original articles, research articles, case reports, case series, and guidelines, then these were subdivided into different chapters according to the system involvement. The goal of the book is to provide the readers with an understanding of the etiology, pathogenesis, genetics, cardiac outcomes, feeding issues, variable neurological affects, urological presentation, endocrinological disturbances; the experience with growth hormone therapy for short stature in Noonan syndrome. We will emphasize to the readers that some individuals with NS can present a mild presentation and at many times without all the above mentioned clinical features. In order to study well the course of the development of this rare entity, I had to review a large volume of articles and original research papers but missed having the authority of a textbook on NS. Also, compounding was the fact about the paucity of long-term data on some of the rare complications of NS. We believe that there is a deficiency and knowledge gap in the process of proper diagnosis of Noonan syndrome and hence came up with the concept and proposal for the book. The authors are international experts in their respective specialties of as pediatric endocrinology, pediatric cardiology, genetics, pediatric urology, anesthesiology, hematology, oncology, pediatric gastroenterology, and dentistry. Furthermore, the team of authors provided an interdisciplinary approach which became essential to review the recently updated publications and write 9 comprehensive chapters encompassing the epidemiology, etiology, diagnosis, and treatment of clinical aspects of Noonan syndrome.

Noonan syndrome is characterized by typical facies, short stature, congenital heart disease, pulmonary valve stenosis, hypertrophic cardiomyopathy and developmental delay of variable degree, webbed neck, chest wall deformities, superior pectus carinatum and inferior pectus excavatum, cryptorchidism, varied coagulation defects, lymphatic dysplasias, and ocular abnormalities. Majority of these were seen in some of the other well-described RASopathies as well. Thus the differential diagnosis includes Costello syndrome, cardiofaciocutaneous syndrome (CFCS), fetal hydantoin syndrome, LEOPARD Lentigines, electrocardiographic (conduction abnormalities), ocular (hypertelorism), pulmonary (stenosis), various short stature and deafness syndrome, disorders of sex development, XO/XY mosaicism, Turner syndrome, neurofibromatosis type 1, and *SPRED1* spectrum [4, 5].

The first published study on Noonan syndrome was in 1962 when Dr. Jacqueline Noonan Pediatric Cardiology from University of Kentucky published the first cases [6, 7]. There were case reports of Noonan syndrome like phenotype even before Dr. Noonan's first description. In 2001 the first report of gene mutation resulting in Noonan syndrome was described by Drs. Trataglia and Gelb of Mount Sinai School of Medicine, New York [8]. Since then there have been hundreds of publications on NS or other RASopathies every year and this text book's primary objective is to bring most of the data and publications together in one reference.

The book will start with the chapter on phenotypic variations and molecular genetics of NS as genetic testing is becoming widely utilized to early and efficient diagnosis as well as to establish a genotype-phenotype correlation. Mutations causing Noonan syndrome alter the genes encoding for the proteins within the RAS/MAPK pathway involved with this pathway which is very similar to the mechanism causing other RASopathies (see Fig. 1). Most of the genes play an important role in a variety of cellular functions including proliferation, migration, cell fate determination, and cell death. At this point there does not seem to be a clear-cut genotype-phenotype correlation but certainly some gene mutations do have a phenotypic predisposition or a salient feature, which is covered in this chapter. Mutations in the *PTPN11* gene are present in nearly 50% of patients with NS [8]. Several other genes have been associated with NS and other RASopathies including *KRAS, SOS1, RAF1, BRAF, SHOC2, NRAS, MEK1, RIT1,* and *CBL. SOS1* mutations are reported in approximately 13%, *RAF1* and *RIT1* each in 5%, and *KRAS* in fewer than 5%. Less than 1% of cases of Noonan syndrome are due to pathogenic *NRAS, BRAF,* and *MAP2K1* gene mutations. Several additional genes associated with a Noonan syndrome-like phenotype in fewer than 10 individuals have been identified. Aggregate genetic testing can diagnose up to approximately 70% of the Noonan syndrome leaving another 30% having an unidentified genetic makeup which remains to be elucidated. The risk in a sibling of a proband

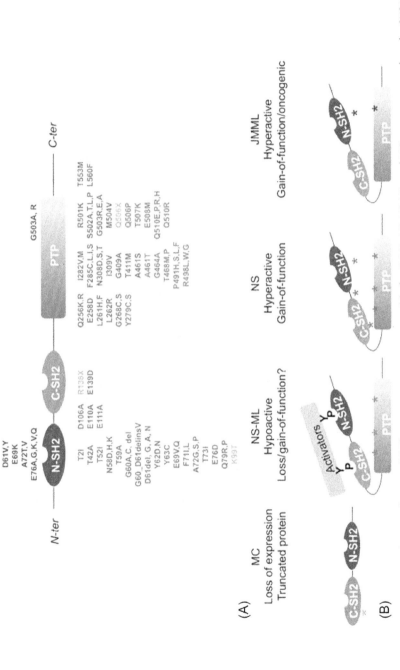

Figure 1 SHP2 mutations in human diseases. (A) The main mutations responsible for JMML, NS, NS-ML, and MC are represented on the SHP2 structure. For MC, note that only missense and nonsense mutations are shown, other mutations (frameshifts, deletion in the noncoding sequence, etc.) being responsible for MC (adapted from NSEuroNet Database, https://nseuronet.com/php/ and https://www.ncbi.nlm.nih.gov/clinvar/PTPN11). (B) Functional consequences of SHP2 mutations. MC-associated mutations result in truncated protein or loss of expression. NS-ML-causing mutations reduce the catalytic activity of SHP2 but may increase its binding affinity for its activator and/or favor its open conformation. NS- and JMML-linked mutations increase SHP2's enzymatic activity and/or abrogate the inhibitory constraints, thereby activating/hyperactivating the phosphatase. *(Reproduced with permission from Elsevier reference Tajan M, de Rocca Serra A, Valet P, Edouard T, Yart A. SHP2 sails from physiology to pathology. Eur J Med Genet 2015;58(10):509–25.)*

depends on the genetic status of the parents. If a parent is affected, the risk is 50%. When the parents are clinically unaffected, the risk to the siblings of a proband appears to be low (<1%). Each child of an individual with Noonan syndrome has a 50% chance of inheriting the pathogenic variant.

Chapter 2 would aim at examining in detail the recent advances in understanding and treating short stature in Noonan Syndrome, as well as the latest progress in GH-dependent signaling pathways involved in short stature. At the time of the birth the weight and length are normal. In the first postnatal life the height begins to dip down and hence short stature is one of the most frequent clinical manifestations of Noonan Syndrome present in approximately 80% of individuals [9]. Studies have reported that the mean final height is usually around 150–152 cm in female and 160–162 cm in males. These final heights have been reported to be even lower in other countries such as Brazil and Japan. In 2007 the U.S. Food and Drug Administration approved treatment of short stature caused by Noonan Syndrome with recombinant growth hormone in doses up to 66 µg/kg/day or 0.46 mg/kg/week. It has been reported that the additional height gain after growth hormone therapy is small, ranging from +0.8 to +1.4 SDS increase, which translates into a final height gain of 5–10 cm at the end of therapy. However, growth hormone treatment for Noonan Syndrome is still controversial and not readily approved by healthcare insurance companies. Also, there are no guidelines for increased cancer surveillance while using growth hormone in most patients with Noonan syndrome, but your clinical decision making is required on individual case basis and what type of mutation they may carry.

One of Noonan syndrome's important characteristics is the presence of heart anomalies. The natural history and outcomes of the congenital heart defects in individuals with Noonan syndrome are different from without the syndrome. Most notable cardiac lesions include pulmonary stenosis associated with dysplastic pulmonary valves; patent foramen ovale and pulmonary stenosis are described in Chapter 3. Altogether 70%–80% of NS individuals have cardiac defects. Pulmonary valve stenosis which has been classically known to be associated with NS is also the most common in about 50%. But children with NS also have other cardiac defects such as atrial septal defect (ASD) in ~20% and then followed by hypertrophic cardiomyopathy (HCM) in about 15%. *PTPN11* gene mutations which account for about 50% of NS have a predilection toward PS and ASD but rarely toward the development of HCM or coarctation of aorta. *RAF1*, *BRAF1*, and *RIT1* mutations have HCM as major feature in NS. The valvular defect of PS in majority remains mild without progression and likely from dysplastic valve. At least one-third patients respond well to balloon angioplasty requiring reintervention in remaining two-third patients. Majority of children with NS are treated with growth hormone therapy to treat their short stature, which warrants regular cardiac surveillance. Growth hormone therapy has a growth-promoting effect on the cardiac musculature and raises a concern on the evolution of HCM in NS. Growth hormone therapy is considered safe to be used from a cardiac standpoint. A detailed cardiac evaluation is necessary and all children with cardiac defects need to cleared and then followed while on growth hormone therapy. In more than half of the patients, HCM is mild with rare progression and favorable prognosis. Other cardiac lesions found in Noonan syndrome are patent ductus arteriosus (PDA) and tetralogy of Fallot. Some of the left-sided anatomic obstruction can occur at the valvular or supravalvular level in the subaortic position as a result of left atrioventricular valve abnormalities or as coarctation of the aortic. Interestingly, the subgroup of patients with Noonan syndrome and aortic coarctation demonstrates male preponderance. Noonan syndrome could present a challenge to an experienced cardiac anesthesiologist and should get a comprehensive preoperative workup and intraoperative monitoring.

Chapter 4 would focus on the various endocrinological expressions or variations seen in NS. The hypothalamic/pituitary/gonadal or adrenal axis in individuals with NS exists has not been studied or reported in literature. Primary gonadal failure relates to cryptorchidism, but perhaps caused delayed puberty, oligospermia, and azoospermia leading to male infertility. The etiology of pubertal delay is not well elucidated but has been reported in both genders when compared to the general population. The mean age of children with NS entering puberty is approximately between 13 and 14 years for females or 13.5–14.5 years for males and [10]. Interestingly, with the exception of delayed puberty, females with NS seem to be spared from gonadal disruptions [10].

Noonan syndrome is associated with congenital abnormalities affecting the genitourinary system. The pathophysiology for most of the urological conditions affecting Noonan syndrome will be addressed in Chapter 5 along with reviewing the surgical techniques being used for cryptorchidism. The patients with cryptorchidism should be referred to a pediatric urologist or an adult urologist depending on the age of the patient for further evaluation and management. Historically, treatment for cryptorchidism was recommended between 1 and 2 years of age based on morphological changes seen on testicular biopsies of undescended testis found on electron microscopy.

However, current guidelines recommend intervention to be done early between 6 and 12 months of age. The treatment options include both medical and surgical modalities. However, medical therapy with human chorionic gonadotropin (HCG) or gonadotropin releasing hormone (GnRH) has a success rate of less than 25% depending on the location of the undescended testis. In this chapter the authors will discuss the diagnosis, use of surgical modalities for cryptorchidism, and other associated genitourinary abnormalities. The renal anomalies associated with Noonan syndrome include a solitary kidney, hydronephrosis, and duplicated renal collecting systems, which can occur in 10%–11% of children. During the pregnancy prenatal period, up to 20% of the Noonan syndrome cases are associated with pelviectasis, hydronephrosis, and renal enlargement. The urinary bladder abnormalities such as urachal cysts associated with Noonan syndrome are rare.

In clinical practice, a large majority of infants with NS encounter feeding difficulties. Again, there is very limited data available in literature regarding gastrointestinal issues in patients with NS or other RASopathies. In this textbook we have dedicated Chapter 6, which compiles the data that were available. The mechanisms that could lead to feeding difficulties in infants with NS could be manifold such as dental and mandibular malformations, gastro-esophageal reflux disease or GERD, abnormal gastro-duodenal motility, and increased incidence of gastrointestinal structural anomalies such as midgut malrotation and hiatal hernia. Birth weight is usually normal in NS and may even be increased due to edema. Majority of infants with NS can then present with failure to thrive caused by feeding difficulties such as poor suck, prolonged feeding times, and recurrent vomiting [11, 12]. A large majority of infants with Noonan syndrome encounter feeding difficulties. In NS there is a very high incidence of malocclusion, high arch palate, micrognathia, enamel hypoplasia leading to feeding difficulties, labial hypotonia, gingival inflammation, and oro-dental malformations. The oral lesions may lead to feeding difficulties due to poor suck, poor latching to breast and bottle during infancy, and poor mastication after dentition has occurred. The distribution of these anomalies in Noonan syndrome patients is not uniform and these may or may not be associated cardiac, so they become a difficult task for early identification and treatment. Chapter 6 is an effort to discuss this poorly understood association of NS and to focus on early detection and intervention of feeding issues and other GI manifestations.

Then Chapter 7 deals with the developmental and neurological features of Noonan syndrome. As you will learn that children with Noonan syndrome are more likely to develop a variety of neurological complications such as developmental delay, seizure disorders, cerebrovascular abnormalities, ocular problems, hearing loss, hypotonia, peripheral neuropathy, hypermobility of joints craniosynostosis, increase in incidence of hydrocephalus, and Arnold Chiari Malformations. Most of these findings are poorly understood and pediatricians should be aware of this higher risk in NS and evaluate early for such neurological symptoms. Although most patients with NS have normal intelligence, about one-third of affected persons have a mild intellectual disability, some have learning difficulties, language impairments, psychological and behavioral problems, such as stubbornness, irritability, and poor self-esteem. This variability is likely related to the patient's specific genetic mutation. These children need early occupational therapy and physiotherapy to improve outcomes.

Chapter 8 is regarding the oncological predispositions and coagulation factor deficiency in Noonan Syndrome. The authors report that the prevalence of bleeding in patients with Noonan Syndrome could range up to 90% depending upon the various methodologies used for diagnosis [13]. Noonan syndrome carries a higher risk of Factor XI deficiency and thrombocytopenia. Other factor deficiencies seen in NS are Factor XII and Factor VIII, respectively, which are also seen in combination with Factor XI deficiency. Early screening for bleeding diathesis is really critical for prevention of morbidity and mortality. Patients with Noonan Syndrome undergo more than average surgical procedure and their risk of bleeding is greater. Clotting and platelet defects considerably restrict the possible analgesic and anesthetic options in patients with Noonan syndrome. The management of patients with Noonan syndrome can be quite complicated due to presentation of multiple deficiencies in a patient. Also, Noonan syndrome with certain *PTPN11* and *KRAS* gene mutations results in an increased childhood malignancy risk than the general population. At high risk are particularly the hematological malignancies such as JMML and some of these processes can start in the early childhood years. Some oncology groups have recommended cancer surveillance from the time of birth or diagnosis to until age 5 years. Certain benign lesions such as giant cell tumors are also associated to occur with *PTPN11* and *SOS1* mutations. Growth hormone therapy is frequently used in children with Noonan syndrome for treatment of short stature. Growth hormone therapy can theoretically increase cancer risk. The children with increased predisposition or high risk for the development of malignancies will need regular monitoring and surveillance. The decision to treat NS children with the high risk *PTPN11* or *KRAS* gene mutations should be done on an individual basis [14]. There have been NS cases of increase in various tumor size growth while they were receiving growth hormone therapy [15].

In Chapter 9 the author will discuss the perioperative considerations in Noonan syndrome as these children with congenital heart defects, chest deformity, cryptorchidism, hematological disorders, facial dysmorphology, and airway anomalies are associated with increased risk of complications from various surgical, anesthetic procedures and anesthetic agents. They also undergo repeated surgical procedures, which further increases the risk of complications. Noonan syndrome is also associated with intellectual deficits and repeated exposure to anesthetics can potentially have an effect on intellectual development, much of which is unknown. In this chapter the commonly reported anesthetic and perioperative complications in Noonan syndrome are discussed, which the anesthesiologist, surgeons, urologist, cardiologist, and endocrinologist need to be aware of while preparing these patients for surgical procedures.

The last but not the least Chapter 10 addresses the many oral and dental manifestations have been associated with NS, which are similar to the GI issues that occur together with each other but sometimes separately from the other general manifestations. The most commonly seen oral manifestations include maxillio-mandibular discrepancies, high arch palate, micrognathia, malocclusion to name a few and along with other dental anomalies. As there are so many of these abnormalities which could be present in NS, it is imperative for hygienists, therapists, dental and medical professionals to understand the nature of these dental oro-facial features to aid in the correct diagnosis and appropriate management.

Of foremost importance are the contributions which have been made by therapists, physician, nurses, healthcare providers, geneticists, molecular scientists, and researchers for their contributions for the exploration of knowledge of Noonan syndrome. The foundation of this book is based upon the countless articles and manuscript of research in the various specialties and fields encompassing Noonan syndrome. I am forever indebted to the authors for the vast effort, resources, and time that they had put in writing these detailed chapters. A work of such nature on this subject has not been undertaken in the past. I take great honor to say that all of the authors are national experts in their respective fields and have spent years taking of care of children with Noonan syndrome. The book intends to provide readers with a comprehensive review covering various aspects such as genetics, diagnosis, cardiac malformations, hematological manifestations, complications from anesthesia along with the experience of growth hormone use in Noonan

Syndrome. This book would not have been possible for the countless and selfless effort put in by expert authors in order to undertake this extraordinary effort. I think the real joy for me was to work with the experts and have an opportunity to present to the learners and readers the results of this comprehensive and detailed work on Noonan syndrome. This effort will come to fruition when we have spread the awareness of Noonan syndrome across the world and the children will receive the rightful care at the right age. I hope that you would read this book to the end and will find that the content was helpful in enhancing your knowledge and skills. I am glad to say that on the date today we have concluded this esteemed book project with the hopes that this shall usher further research, development, and help spread the knowledge to any learner keen on Noonan syndrome.

Yours Sincerely,

Amrit P.S. Bhangoo, MD
Editor & Pediatric Endocrinologist
May 29th 2018

REFERENCES

[1] Romano AA, Blethen SL, Dana K, Noto RA. Growth hormone treatment in Noonan syndrome: the National Cooperative Growth Study experience. J Pediatr 1996;128(5 Pt 2):S18–21.

[2] Osio D, Dahlgren J, Wikland KA, Westphal O. Improved final height with long-term growth hormone treatment in Noonan syndrome. Acta Paediatr 2005;94(9):1232–7.

[3] van der Burgt I. Noonan syndrome. Orphanet J Rare Dis 2007;2:4.

[4] Bhambhani V, Muenke M. Noonan syndrome. Am Fam Physician 2014;89(1):37–43.

[5] Cao H, Alrejaye N, Klein OD, Goodwin AF, Oberoi S. A review of craniofacial and dental findings of the RASopathies. Orthod Craniofacial Res 2017;20(Suppl 1):32–8. https://doi.org/10.1111/ocr.12144.

[6] Noonan JA, Ehmke DA. Associated non cardiac malformations in children with congenital heart disease. J Pediatr 1963;63:468–70.

[7] Noonan JA. Hypertelorism with Turner phenotype. A new syndrome with associated congenital heart disease. Am J Dis Child 1968;116(4):373–80.

[8] Tartaglia M, Mehler EL, Goldberg R, Zampino G, Brunner HG, Kremer H, et al. Mutations in PTPN11, encoding the protein tyrosine phosphatase SHP-2, cause Noonan syndrome. Nat Genet 2001;29(4):465–8.

[9] Tartaglia M, Gelb BD, Zenker M. Noonan syndrome and clinically related disorders. Best Pract Res Clin Endocrinol Metab 2011;25(1):161–79.

[10] Romano AA, Allanson JE, Dahlgren J, Gelb BD, Hall B, Pierpont ME, et al. Noonan syndrome: clinical features, diagnosis, and management guidelines. Pediatrics 2010;126 (4):746–59.

[11] Sharland M, Burch M, McKenna WM, Paton MA. A clinical study of Noonan syndrome. Arch Dis Child 1992;67(2):178–83.

[12] Shaw AC, Kalidas K, Crosby AH, Jeffery S, Patton MA. The natural history of Noonan syndrome: a long-term follow-up study. Arch Dis Child 2007;92(2):128–32. https://doi.org/10.1136/adc.2006.104547. Epub 2006 Sep 21.

[13] BB J, DJ D. Bleeding disorders in Noonan syndrome. Pediatr Blood Cancer 2012;58 (2):167–72.

[14] Raman S, Grimberg A, Waguespack SG, Miller BS, Sklar CA, Meacham LR, et al. Risk of neoplasia in pediatric patients receiving growth hormone therapy—a report from the Pediatric Endocrine Society Drug and Therapeutics Committee. J Clin Endocrinol Metab 2015;100(6):2192–203.

[15] McWilliams GD, SantaCruz K, Hart B, Clericuzio C. Occurrence of DNET and other brain tumors in Noonan syndrome warrants caution with growth hormone therapy. Am J Med Genet A 2016;170(1):195–201.

FURTHER READING

[16] Tajan M, de Rocca Serra A, Valet P, Edouard T, Yart A. SHP2 sails from physiology to pathology. Eur J Med Genet 2015;58(10):509–25.

CHAPTER 1

Noonan Syndrome: Phenotypic Variations and Molecular Genetics

Neda Zadeh
Genetics Center, Orange, CA, United States
CHOC Children's Hospital, Orange, CA, United States

Abstract

Noonan syndrome is a genetic multisystemic disorder with a prevalence of 1 in 1000–2500 newborns. This condition is characterized by dysmorphic features, developmental delay, short stature, congenital heart disease, lymphatic malformations, genitourinary anomalies, and bleeding difficulties. Mutations that cause Noonan syndrome alter genes encoding proteins with a role in the RAS/MAPK pathway. Medical management guidelines have been developed for this condition and molecular genetic testing is available diagnostically and may provide further aid in long medical management and prognosis (Roberts et al. [5]).

Keywords: Noonan syndrome, RASopathy, Ras-MAPK, PTPN11

Abbreviations

CFC	cardiofaciocutaneous syndrome
NS	Noonan syndrome
NT	nuchal translucency
RAS/MAPK pathway	Ras/mitogen-activated protein kinase pathway

INTRODUCTION

Noonan syndrome (NS) is a multisystemic genetic condition that occurs in 1:1000–2500 live births. An incorrect term utilized to describe this condition is the "male Turner syndrome" which incorrectly implied that this condition would not be observed in females. As Noonan syndrome is an autosomal dominant disorder, it is observed in both males and females [1]. Characteristic features include short stature, congenital cardiac defects, dysmorphic features, and variable developmental delay and learning difficulties. Other features include sternal abnormalities, genitourinary abnormalities, lymphatic dysplasia, and coagulation defects. Hypertrophic cardiomyopathy can also be observed in approximately 20%–30% of patients. In addition, individuals with Noonan syndrome have an increased risk of developing cancer. Noonan syndrome is diagnosed clinically, with

Noonan Syndrome
https://doi.org/10.1016/B978-0-12-815348-2.00010-4

the average age at diagnosis of 9 years [2]. Molecular testing is becoming much more utilized to provide diagnostic confirmation as well as to attempt to provide genotype-phenotype correlation. Mutations that cause Noonan syndrome alter genes encoding proteins within the RAS/MAPK pathway, which plays a role in a variety of functions including proliferation, migration, cell fate determination, and senescence [3]. This pathway also participates in early and late developmental process including organogenesis, morphology determination, and growth [4]. Heterozygous pathogenic mutations in nine genes account for approximately 75%–80% of all Noonan syndrome cases. Within the past several years, whole exome sequencing has allowed identification of new variants in rare genes [3]. Therefore molecular diagnosis is helpful in diagnostic confirmation and also potentially provides genotype-phenotype correlations and accurate risk assessment [1,5].

RASopathies

The RAS/MAPK pathway is an important signal transduction pathway through which extracellular ligands stimulate cell proliferation, differentiation, survival, and metabolism [5] (Fig. 1). Ligand binding to cell surface receptors causes site-specific phosphorylation within certain cytoplasmic regions. This leads to recruitment of adaptor proteins which form a complex with guanine nucleotide exchange factors that convert inactive RAS-GDP to its active RAS-GTP form. This activated form of RAS protein then activates the RAF-MEK-ERK cascade through a series of phosphorylation events. The end product of activated ERK then enters the nucleus to alter gene transcription [5]. Due to its role in signal transduction, signal through the RAS/MAPK pathway is normally tightly controlled, with enhanced flow through the pathway contributing to oncogenesis [4].

The RASopathies are a clinically defined group of medical genetic syndromes caused by mutations in genes that encode components or regulators of the RAS/MAPK pathway as described before [6]. Genetic conditions included in the group of RASopathies include Noonan syndrome, Costello syndrome, cardiofaciocutaneous (CFC) syndrome, Legius syndrome, Noonan syndrome with multiple lentigines (formerly LEOPARD syndrome), and capillary malformation-ateriovenous malformation syndrome (CM-AVM) [6].

All the known genes associated with Noonan syndrome encode proteins integral to the above described pathway [5,6]. As the other RASopathy conditions are associated with genes that are integral to the function of the RAS/MAPK pathway, many clinical features may be similar or overlapping, often

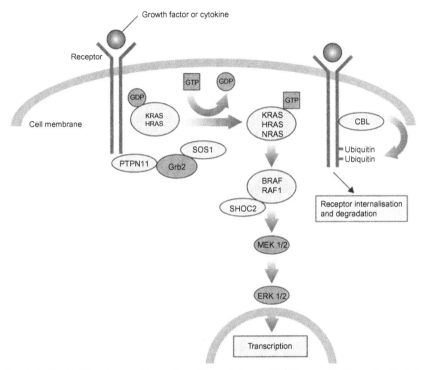

Fig. 1 RAS/MAPK pathway. *(Reproduced from Roberts AE, Allanson JE, Tartaglia M, Gelb BD. Noonan syndrome. Lancet 2013;381(9863):333–42.)*

making clinical diagnoses difficult and underlying the diagnostic aid of molecular testing.

CLINICAL FEATURES OF NOONAN SYNDROME

Noonan syndrome should be suspected in individuals with the following key features (modified from Allanson et al. [1]):

- *Characteristic facial features.* Facial features of patients with Noonan syndrome show considerable differences depending on the age of the patient, being more striking during infancy and adolescence, and more subtle in adulthood [2] (Fig. 2).

    During infancy, the head can appear relatively large with a tall forehead, hypertelorism with downslanting palpebral fissures, low-set posteriorly rotated ears with thickened helix, deeply grooved philtrum with high wide peaks to the vermillion border of the upper lip [1,2,5]. Eyes are often prominent with full or ptotic eyelids. There is usually a depressed

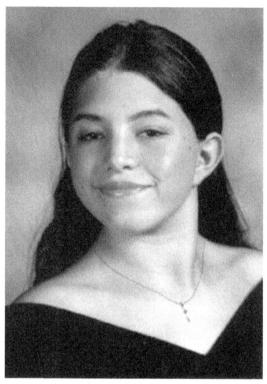

Fig. 2 Eighteen-year-old young lady with Noonan syndrome. *(Reproduced from Noonan JA. Noonan syndrome and related disorders. Prog Pediatr Cardiol 2005;20(2):177–85. https://doi.org//10.1016/j.ppedcard.2005.04.008, Elsevier.)*

nasal root, wide base, and bulbous tip. The hair can by wispy during the toddler years [1,2].

In childhood there is often myopathic facies with decreased facial expression. By adolescence the facial shape resembles an inverted triangle with a wide forehead and tapered chin. Eyes often become less prominent, and the neck lengthens, which may accentuate nuchal webbing. The hair is often curly or wooly [2].

In adults there are prominent nasolabial folds and skin can often have a transparent and prematurely wrinkled appearance [1,2].

Ocular anomalies can include strabismus, refractive errors, amblyopia, and nystagmus in up to 95% of patients. There are a few case reports of keratoconus and Axenfeld anomaly. Iris color can be lighter than what is typically expected for ethnic background [1,2].

- *Short stature.* Birth weight and length are generally normal with signs of postnatal growth failure noted by 12 months of age, which tends to track along the 3rd percentile from early childhood until puberty. The prevalence of short stature in Noonan syndrome is most notable during pubertal ages, often with delayed bone age. Often, catch-up growth can occur during later teen years, with prolonged growth into the 20s that is possible. Growth hormone deficiency, neurosecretory dysfunction, and growth hormone resistance have been described. Growth hormone treatment data can be difficult to compare due to differing protocols and outcome criteria [5]. However, short stature due to Noonan syndrome is an FDA-approved indication for growth hormone treatment. The final adult height can approach the lower limit of normal with 161–167 cm in males and 150–155 cm in females [1,2]. Specific growth curves exist and can be accessed under Noonan syndrome clinical management guidelines on the RASopathies network web page (https://rasopathiesnet.org).
- *Congenital cardiac defect.* Noonan syndrome is the second most common syndromic cause of congenital heart disease [7]. The most common abnormalities include pulmonary valve stenosis often with dysplasia (20%–60%), hypertrophic cardiomyopathy (20%–30%), and secundum atrial septal defect (6%–10%). Ventricular septal defect, peripheral pulmonary stenosis, atrioventricular canal, aortic stenosis, mitral valve abnormalities, aortic coarctation, and coronary artery anomalies have also been observed [5]. Cardiomyopathy usually presents early in life with a median age of diagnosis of 5 months [8].
- *Developmental delay.* Early developmental milestones may be delayed due to findings of hypotonia and resultant increased joint laxity. Most children with Noonan syndrome sit unassisted around 10 months and walk at 21 months [1]. Approximately 25% of children have learning difficulties with 10%–15% requiring special education setting, with others having normal intelligence with IQ ranges between 70 and 120 [5]. The first word is spoken at 15 months with two word phrases emerging between 31 and 32 months. Articulation may be an issue for many children, but generally this responds well to speech therapy. Behavioral issues or psychopathology has not been generally observed.
- *Broad or webbed neck.* Many of the postnatally observed features of Noonan syndrome can be secondary to consequences of *in utero* lymphatic obstruction or dysfunction [5]. These can include findings of a broad or webbed neck and prominence of the trapezius and low posterior hairline [2].

- *Unusual chest shape (superior pectus carinatum and inferior pectus excavatum) with widely spaced nipples.* These features are also secondary to *in utero* lymphatic obstruction.
- *Cryptorchidism in males and genitourinary anomalies.* Renal abnormalities are noted in approximately 11% of patients, with the most common anomaly being dilatation of the renal pelvis [5]. Duplex collecting systems, renal hypoplasia, unilateral renal agenesis, and bilateral cysts with scarring have also been reported. Unilateral or bilateral cryptorchidism is observed in 60%–80% of affected males. Primary Sertoli cell dysfunction is suggested to cause male gonadal dysfunction rather than cryptorchidism [5]. Puberty is generally delayed with a mean age of menarche of 14.6 years in females. Fertility is expected to be normal in females, in males complications can arise from undetected/untreated cryptorchidism and Sertoli cell dysfunction [5].
- *Coagulation defects.* Most individuals with Noonan syndrome have a history of some form of abnormal bleeding or bruising. Coagulopathy can manifest as a spectrum from severe surgical hemorrhage to clinically mild bruising [1]. Aspirin therapy is generally recommended to be avoided in individuals with Noonan syndrome.
- *Lymphatic abnormalities.* The pathogenesis of Noonan syndrome may be partially due to jugular lymphatic obstruction in utero. Findings of cryptorchidism, along with other features previously described such as webbed neck, widely spaced nipples, low set and angulated ears are postulated to be due to tissue disruption or displacement by lymphedema during embryonic development [2].

  Fewer than 20% of patients with Noonan syndrome have a lymphatic abnormality. Peripheral lymphedema (usually involving the dorsal limb) can be observed during infancy and may resolve during the first few years of life, with occasional representation during adulthood. Less commonly observed is hydrops fetalis, pulmonary, testicular or intestinal lymphangiectasia, chylous effusion of the pleural space and peritoneum, and aplasia or absence of the thoracic duct [5].

Additional findings include café au lait macules, lentigines, and keratosis pilaris. Approximately 5% of patients may have hypothyroidism [2]. There have also been single case reports in the medical literature of autoimmune dysfunction including vasculitis, vitiligo, and anterior uveitis [2]. There is an increased risk for certain hematological cancers compared to that of the general population, including juvenile myelomonocytic leukemia (JMML) which tends to run a more benign course, acute myelogenous leukemia (AML) and B-cell acute lymphoblastic leukemia (B-ALL). Cases of solid tumors such as embryonal rhabdomyosarcoma have been reported as well as glial tumors [1,5]. During infancy, transient myeloproliferative disorders can be more common. Lastly, advanced paternal age has been seen in association with many of the observed simplex cases of RASopathies, including Noonan syndrome.

Prenatal Findings

Noonan syndrome may present prenatally with abnormal ultrasound findings which can often be nonspecific and do not correlate with the severity of the postnatal phenotype [9]. Ultrasound findings can include polyhydramnios, increased nuchal translucency (NT) measurement during the first trimester, cystic hygroma, relative macrocephaly, pleural and pericardial effusion, ascites as well as fetal cardiac and renal anomalies. A common prenatal indicator of lymphatic dysfunction that can be seen on prenatal ultrasound is a cystic hygroma [2]. Regression of the cystic hygroma prior to the mid-second trimester is associated with better prognosis, however some done not resolve and can progress to hydrops [2]. In chromosomally normal fetuses with an increased NT measurement, it is estimated that 5%–15% may have Noonan syndrome [1,10]. As mentioned previously, many of the postnatally observed features of Noonan syndrome can be secondary to consequences of in utero lymphatic obstruction or dysfunction [5].

ESTABLISHING THE DIAGNOSIS OF NOONAN SYNDROME

The diagnosis of Noonan syndrome can be made clinically as outlined before and often includes identification of a heterozygous pathogenic mutation in a known associated gene. Molecular diagnostic testing can be performed by serial single gene testing, by a multigene panel, or for rarer forms of Noonan syndrome, may be detected by whole exome sequencing [1]. Approximately 50% of individuals with Noonan syndrome have a pathogenic missense point mutation in the *PTPN11* gene. Therefore single gene testing can be elected for this gene with reflex to a larger panel.

MOLECULAR GENETICS

Noonan syndrome is caused by a gain-of-function mechanism. Heterozygous pathogenic mutations in *PTPN11, KRAS, SOS1, RAF1, SHOC2,*

NRAS, *CBL*, *BRAF*, and *MAP2K1* account for approximately 75%–80% of all Noonan syndrome cases [3]. Additionally known associated genes include *RIT1*, *PPP1CB*, *SOS2*, and *LTRZ1*.

GENOTYPE-PHENOTYPE CORRELATIONS

PTPN11

The *PTPN11* gene (OMIM *176876) is composed of two tandemly arranged aminoterminal SH-2 domains: N-SH2 and C-SH2, a phosphotyrosine phosphatase (PTP) domain and a carboxy-terminal tail. This gene encodes SHP-2 (Src homology 2 domain-containing protein tyrosine phosphatase [PTP]) which activates the RAS/MAPK pathway. Approximately 50% of patients with Noonan syndrome have a heterozygous gain-of-function mutation in this gene [1,5]. Thus mutations in this gene result in the constitutive activation of the RAS/MAPK pathway in the absence of growth factors [2,11]. In *PTPN11* there are mutation hotspots in exons 3, 8, 9, and 13 which are mostly located in or around the interacting surfaces of the N-SH2 and PTP functional domains [2].

Heterozygous mutations in *PTPN11* can be seen more frequently in association with pulmonary stenosis, short stature, easy bruising with factor VIII deficiency, pectus deformity, and typical facial appearance as described previously [2]. The majority of patients with mutations in this gene exhibit some degree of cognitive impairment. Furthermore, de novo mutations in this gene can be seen more frequently with advanced paternal age or are paternal in origin.

Ptpn11 mouse model exhibited increased ERK activation in response to growth hormone, thus inhibiting growth hormone-induced IGF-1 release through RAS/ERK hyperactivation, which is a mechanism that may contribute to observed growth restriction and short stature. Inhibition of ERK1/2 activation in mouse models resulted in an increase of IGF-1 levels in vitro and in vivo, leading to significant growth improvement in *ptpn11* knock out mouse model [11a].

Patients with *PTPN11*-associated Noonan syndrome may have normal to increased concentrations of growth hormone and low concentrations of IGF1 demonstrating resistance to growth hormone [5]. Multiple giant cell lesions are associated with both *PTPN11*- or *SOS1*-related Noonan syndrome [5]. These are giant-cell granulomas and bone and joint anomalies that can resemble cherubism [1].

Review of the medical literature has revealed an estimated 3–5 times increased risk of developing cancer in patients with *PTPN11* mutations compared to the general population [5]. Specifically, heterozygous pathogenic variants at codons 61, 71, 72, and 76 are significantly associated with leukemogenesis and identify a subgroup of patients at risk for JMML [1,12].

SOS1

Heterozygous mutations in the *SOS1* gene (OMIM *182530) are the second most common cause of Noonan syndrome accounting for about 10%–13% of cases [1,6]. The protein product of this gene is a regulator for RAS signal transduction. RAS genes in general encode membrane-bound guanine nucleotide binding proteins which function in signal transduction regulating cell growth and differentiation. Therefore the protein product of *SOS1* may act as a positive regulator of RAS by promoting guanine nucleotide exchange (GDP to GTP). Most observed patients with mutations in this gene have typical facial features, cardiac abnormalities, ectodermal abnormalities (sparse eyebrows, hyperkeratosis pilaris, and ulerythema ophryogenes) along with normal development and stature compared to other patients with Noonan syndrome [1–3,13].

RAF1

Heterozygous gain-of-function mutations in *RAF1* (OMIM *164760) account for approximately 4%–5% of patients with Noonan syndrome. This is one of three genes that activate the MEK-ERK cascade. Hypertrophic cardiomyopathy is overrepresented in *RAF1*-related Noonan syndrome (75% of patients) and is most often seen in association with mutations in the Ser259 and Ser621 hotspots. Furthermore, one-third of patients with *RAF1*-related Noonan syndrome can have multiple nevi and/or café au lait macules [1,5].

KRAS

Mutations in *KRAS* (OMIM *190070) are a rare cause of Noonan syndrome, occurring in less than 5% of patients. This gene product also acts as intracellular signal transducers. Patients with mutations in this gene tend to have a less typical phenotype with severe intellectual disability compared to other molecular causes of this condition. Two unrelated individuals with craniosynostosis and *KRAS*-related Noonan syndrome have been reported [1,2,14].

NRAS

Mutations in NRAS (OMIM *164790) have also been found in a very small number of patients with Noonan syndrome. The product of this gene also is part of the RAS protein family. There are currently no established genotype-phenotype correlations [1]. A case report by De Filippi et al. in 2009 described a 2-month-old infant with a heterozygous G13D mutation in NRAS along with characteristic facies, congenital cardiac defect, café au lait macules, and JMML [15].

BRAF, MAP2K1

Mutations in BRAF (MIM *164757) have been reported both in patients with Noonan syndrome as well as another RASopathy: cardiofaciocutaneous syndrome. Approximately less than 2% of patients have BRAF-associated Noonan syndrome. The majority of published patient cases have mutations that cluster in the cysteine-rich domain and in the aminoterminal portion and activation segment of the kinase domain in this gene. Substitutions of residues Gln257 and Glu501 account for approximately 40% of observed mutations (including hotspots in exons 6, 12, and 15) [16]. Phenotype correlations include neonatal growth failure, feeding difficulties, short stature, dolichocephaly, multiple nevi, dark colored lentigines, mild to moderate cognitive impairment, skeletal anomalies, hypotonia, polyhydramnios, and hypertrophic cardiomyopathy [1,5]. It is important to note that sporadic tumors can occur with somatic nucleotide variants in BRAF or MAP2K1 (OMIM *176872) that are not present in the germline. This phenomenon can also be observed for somatic mutations in PTPN11, KRAS, and NRAS. Therefore these individuals would not have NS, nor a hereditary cancer predisposition condition due to absence of the mutation from germline cells.

RIT1

Approximately 5% of patients with Noonan syndrome have pathogenic variants in RIT1 (OMIM *609591) [1]. The product of RIT1 shares homology with other RAS proteins and expression of mutant alleles demonstrate a gain-of-function effect. Approximately 70%–75% of patients with RIT1-related Noonan syndrome have hypertrophic cardiomyopathy, congenital cardiac defects (septal defects and pulmonary valve stenosis), arrhythmia, milder craniofacial features, macrosomia, macrocephaly, generalized skin hyperpigmentation, excess hyperelastic skin along the palms of the hands and soles of the feet, and lymphatic dysplasia. Stature is typically normal, as is intelligence, with learning or intellectual disabilities reported in a minority of patients [15,17].

CBL

Mutations in *CBL* (OMIM *165360) are very infrequently seen in patients with Noonan syndrome (<1%). The protein product of this gene acts as a negative regulator of several receptor protein tyrosine kinase signaling pathways. Martinelli et al. reported four unrelated patients with variable clinical features that were highly consistent with Noonan syndrome with associated mutations in this gene [4]. Another patient cohort reported by Perez et al. involved three unrelated female patients who all developed juvenile myelomonocytic leukemia (JMML) prior to 26 months of life along with findings of microcephaly, postnatal growth restriction, dysmorphic features, and developmental delay [18]. In JMML and other myeloid malignancies, *CBL* mutations generally occurred as acquired homozygous mutations as a result of acquired isodisomy at chromosome 11q23.3 that encompasses the *CBL* locus. Thus in individuals with germline *CBL* pathogenic mutations, it is expected that there may be a congenital predisposition to specific malignancies such as JMML [4].

SHOC2

The *SHOC2* gene (OMIM 602775) encodes a protein of the same name which plays an essential role in the RAS/MAPK pathway regulation. A recurrent *SHOC2* gene mutation, 4A>G (p.Ser2Gly) occurs in a subgroup of patients (5%) with features of Noonan syndrome and additional features of loose anagen hair, skin anomalies (ichthyosis, generalized hyperpigmentation with hyperkeratosis), hypernasal speech, hyperactive behavior, and cardiac septal defects. Loose anagen hair presents with easily pluckable, sparse, thin and slow growing hair with an irregular texture. This is caused by an abnormal hair bulb that lacks inner and outer root sheaths [19].

PPP1CB

Heterozygous mutations in *PPP1CB* (OMIM *600590) have been described in association with Noonan syndrome-like disorder with loose anagen hair. To date, all mutations observed have been identified by whole exome sequencing. This gene is highly expressed in the human brain throughout development. Clinical features include global developmental delay, intellectual disability, congenital cardiac defects, macrocephaly, short stature often due to growth hormone deficiency, and more coarse appearing facial features [19]. Clinical features are quite similar to those observed in patients with *SHOC2* gene mutations. Faint café au lait macules and hyperpigmented lesion as well as reckless were noted without findings of hyperkeratosis [19].

Additional Genes

Additional newly described Noonan syndrome causative genes include *SOS2* (OMIM *601247) and *LZTR1* (OMIM *600574). *SOS2* encodes a RAS guanine nucleotide exchange factor, with all described mutations causing enhanced signaling from RAS to ERK in the RAS/MAPK pathway [20]. All reported patients in the medical literature have features that are almost identical to those observed in patients with *SOS1* mutations, including ectodermal abnormalities especially ulerythema ophryogenes which was the most prominently observed finding, followed by typical facial features, cardiac defects including septal defects, coarctation of the aorta, and pulmonary valve stenosis [3,20]. Other ectodermal abnormalities include facial keratosis pilaris and sparse scalp hair [20].

Yamamoto et al. also reported five unrelated families with five different rare variants identified by exome sequencing in the Kelch (KT) domain of the *LZTR1* gene to be causative of Noonan syndrome. The majority of patients have typical facial features and cardiac abnormalities including pulmonary stenosis and mitral valve defects. One patient developed multiple schwannomas on the upper extremity [3].

CONCLUSION

The presentation of Noonan syndrome can often be subtle or difficult to diagnose clinically. Genetic testing technology has provided confirmatory diagnosis as well as discovered new implicated genes and phenotypes. As this is a multisystemic condition, this underlines the necessity for long-term follow-up and multidisciplinary involvement.

REFERENCES

[1] Allanson JE, Roberts AE. Noonan syndrome. In: Adam MP, Ardinger HH, Pagon RA, et al., editors. GeneReviews® [Internet]. Seattle, WA: University of Washington; 1993–2018. 2001 Nov 15 [Updated 2016 Feb 25]. Available from:https://www.ncbi.nlm.nih.gov/books/NBK1124/.

[2] Allanson JE. Management of genetic syndromes. 3rd ed; 2010. p. 569–86.

[3] Yamamoto GL, Aguena M, Gos M, et al. Rare variants in SOS2 and LZTR1 are associated with Noonan syndrome. J Med Genet 2015;52:413–21.

[4] Martinelli S, De Luca A, Stellacci E, et al. Heterozygous germline mutations in the CBL tumor-suppressor gene cause a Noonan syndrome-like phenotype. Am J Hum Genet 2010;87:250–7.

[5] Roberts AE, Allanson JE, Tartaglia M, Gelb BD. Noonan syndrome. Lancet 2013;381 (9863):333–42.

[6] Rauen KA. The RASopathies. Annu Rev Genomics Hum Genet 2013;14:355–69.

[7] Marino B, Digilio MC, Toscano A, Giannotti A, Dallapiccola B. Congenital heart disease in children with Noonan syndrome: an expanded cardiac spectrum with high prevalence of atrioventricular canal. J Pediatr 1999;135:703–6.

[8] Wilkinson JD, Lowe AM, Salbert BA, et al. Outcomes in children with Noonan syndrome and hypertrophic cardiomyopathy: a study from the Pediatric Cardiomyopathy Registry. Am Heart J 2012;164:442–8.

[9] Hakami F, Dillon MW, Lebo M, Mason-Suares H. Retrospective study of prenatal ultrasound findings in newborns with a Noonan spectrum disorder. Prenat Diagn 2016;36:418–23.

[10] Bakker M, Pajkrt E, Bilardo CM. Increased nuchal translucency with normal karyotype and anomaly scan: what next? Best Pract Res Clin Obstet Gynaecol 2014;28:355–66.

[11] Sakamoto K, Imamura T, Asai D, et al. Acute lymphoblastic leukemia developing in a patient with Noonan syndrome harboring a PTPN11 germline mutation. J Pediatr Hematol Oncol 2014;36:e136–9.

[11a] De Rocca Serra-Nedelec A, Edouard T, Trequer K, Tajan M, Araki T, Dance M, Mus M, Montagner A, Tauber M, Salles JP, Valet P, Neel BG, Raynal P, Yart A. Noonan syndrome causing SHP2 mutations inhibit insulin-like growth factor 1 release via growth hormone-induced ERK hyperactivation, which contributes to short stature. Proc Natl Acad Sci USA 2012;109(11):4257–62.

[12] Niihori T, Aoki Y, Ohashi H, Kurosawa K, Kondoh T, Ishikiriyama S, Kawame H, Kamasaki H, Yamanaka T, Takada F, Nishio K, Sakurai M, Tamai H, Nagashima T, Suzuki Y, Kure S, Fujii K, Imaizumi M, Matsubara Y. Functional analysis of PTPN11/SHP-2 mutants identified in Noonan syndrome and childhood leukemia. J Hum Genet 2005;50:192–202.

[13] Tartaglia M, Pennacchio LA, Zhao C, Yadav KK, Fodale V, Sarkozy A, Pandit B, Oishi K, Martinelli S, Schackwitz W, Ustaszewska A, Martin J, Bristow J, Carta C, Lepri F, Neri C, Vasta I, Gibson K, Curry CJ, Siguero JP, Digilio MC, Zampino G, Dallapiccola B, Bar-Sagi D, Gelb BD. Gain-of-function SOS1 mutations cause a distinctive form of Noonan syndrome. Nat Genet 2007;39:75–9.

[14] Kratz CP, Zampino G, Kriek M, Kant SG, Leoni C, Pantaleoni F, Oudesluys-Murphy AM, Di Rocco C, Kloska SP, Tartaglia M, Zenker M. Craniosynostosis in patients with Noonan syndrome caused by germline KRAS mutations. Am J Med Genet A 2009;149A:1036–40.

[15] De Filippi P, Zecca M, Lisini D, Rosti V, Cagioni C, Carlo-Stella C, Radi O, Veggiotti P, Mastronuzzi A, Acquaviva A, D'Ambrosio A, Locatelli F, Danesino C. Germline mutation of the NRAS gene may be responsible for the development of juvenile myelomonocytic leukaemia. Br J Haematol 2009;147:706–9.

[16] Sarkozy A, Carta C, Moretti S, Zampino G, Digilio MC, Pantaleoni F, Scioletti AP, Esposito G, Cordeddu V, Lepri F, Petrangeli V, Dentici ML, Mancini GM, Selicorni A, Rossi C, Mazzanti L, Marino B, Ferrero GB, Silengo MC, Memo L, Stanzial F, Faravelli F, Stuppia L, Puxeddu E, Gelb BD, Dallapiccola B, Tartaglia M. Germline BRAF mutations in Noonan, LEOPARD, and cardiofaciocutaneous syndromes: molecular diversity and associated phenotypic spectrum. Hum Mutat 2009;30:695–702.

[17] Kouz K, Lissewski C, Spranger S, et al. Genotype and phenotype in patients with Noonan syndrome and a RIT1 mutation. Genet Med 2016;18(12):1226–34.

[18] Perez B, Mechinaud F, Galambrun C, et al. Germline mutations of the CBL gene define a new genetic syndrome with predisposition to juvenile myelomonocytic leukaemia. J Med Genet 2010;47:686–91.

[19] Ma L, Bayram U, McLaughlin HM, et al. *De novo* missense variants in PPP1CB are associated with intellectual disabilities and congenital cardiac disease. Hum Genet 2016;135(12):1399–409.

[20] Cordeddu V, Yin JC, Gunnarsson C, et al. Activating mutations affecting the Dbl homology domain of SOS2 cause Noonan syndrome. Hum Mutat 2015;36:1080–7.

FURTHER READING

[21] Gripp KW, Aldinger KA, Bennett JT, et al. A novel rasopathy caused by recurrent de novo missense mutations in PPP1CB closely resembles Noonan syndrome with loose anagen hair. Am J Med Genet A 2016;170(9):2237–47.

[22] Noonan JA. Noonan syndrome and related disorders. Prog Pediatr Cardiol 2005; 20(2):177–85. https://doi.org/10.1016/j.ppedcard.2005.04.008.

CHAPTER 2

Growth Failure and Experience With Growth Hormone Therapy in Noonan Syndrome

Alexsandra C. Malaquias*, Alexander A.L. Jorge[†]
*Division of Pediatric Endocrinology, Department of Pediatrics, Faculty of Medical Sciences, Santa Casa de Sao Paulo, Sao Paulo, Brazil
[†]Division of Endocrinology-Genetics (LIM/25), Discipline of Endocrinology, Faculty of Medicine, University of Sao Paulo (USP), Sao Paulo, Brazil

Abstract

Noonan syndrome (NS, OMIM 163950) is a frequent autosomal dominant disorder characterized by facial dysmorphisms, short stature, and congenital heart defects. Mutations related to RAS/MAPK (mitogen-activated protein kinase) signaling pathway have shown to be involved in the pathogenesis of NS as well as Noonan-like syndromes (NLS). These mutations are predicted to be gain-of-function defects increasing signaling down the RAS/MAPK pathway. Several hormones act through receptors that stimulate the RAS/MAPK pathway, and therefore, NS and related disorders present implications in different endocrine systems, including the GH/IGF-1 system. Additionally, adult height of NS patients has shown improvement after recombinant human growth hormone (rhGH) treatment. In this chapter, we review the diagnostic, clinical, and molecular aspects of NS and rhGH treatment of short stature in these patients.

Keywords: Noonan syndrome, RASopathies, RAS/MAPK, Short stature, Growth hormone

NOMENCLATURE

A2ML1	alpha-2-macroglobulin-Like 1
BMI	body mass index
BRAF	V-RAF murine sarcoma viral oncogene homolog B1
KRAS	V-KI-Ras2 Kirsten rat sarcoma viral oncogene
LZTR1	leucine zipper-like transcriptional regulator 1
MAP2K1	mitogen-activated protein kinase kinase 1
M-CSF	macrophage colony-stimulating factor
NRAS	neuroblastoma Ras viral oncogene homolog
PTPN11	protein-tyrosine phosphatase, nonreceptor-type, 11
RAF1	V-RAF-1 murine leukemia viral oncogene homolog 1
RANKL	receptor activator of nuclear factor kappa B ligand
RASA2	RAS p21 protein activator 2

Noonan Syndrome
https://doi.org/10.1016/B978-0-12-815348-2.00001-3

RIT1   RIC-like protein without CAAX motif 1
RRAS   related Ras viral oncogene homolog
SGA   small for gestational age
SHOC2   suppressor of clear, *C. elegans*, homolog of
SHP-2   SH2-domains containing tyrosine phosphatase 2
SOS1   son of sevenless, Drosophila, homolog 1
SOS2   son of sevenless, Drosophila, homolog 2

INTRODUCTION

Noonan syndrome (NS, OMIM 163950) is a frequent autosomal dominant disorder characterized by facial dysmorphisms, short stature, and congenital heart defects. It is believed to be one of the most common syndromes with a Mendelian autosomal dominant inheritance pattern and near complete penetrance. The estimated incidence of severely affected individuals is between 1:1000 and 1:2500 [1]. Familial cases are described in approximately 20% of the patients. Maternal transmission is more frequent than paternal, possibly reflecting impaired male fertility due to cryptorchidism [2].

The diagnosis of NS is primarily based on clinical findings. Usually, typical facial features associated with short stature or cardiac malformation prompts the suspicion of NS. Characteristic facial features include a triangular face, low-set posteriorly rotated ears with the thickened helix, ptosis, ocular hypertelorism, down-slanting palpebral fissures, epicanthal fold, deeply grooved philtrum, high-arched palate, and micrognathia. The accurate and straightforward score system proposed by van der Burgt in 1994 is frequently adopted for NS diagnosis [3]. However, establishing the clinical diagnosis can be difficult in patients with mild forms.

The molecular cause of NS was first described in 2001 by Tartaglia et al. who identified heterozygous missense mutations in *PTPN11* gene (OMIM 176876) in patients with NS. *PTPN11* encodes a ubiquitously expressed cytoplasmic protein, SHP-2, which positively regulates signal flux through the RAS/MAPK pathway. Mutations in the *PTPN11* gene are present in nearly 50% of patients with NS [4].

Since then, mutations in *A2ML1, BRAF, CBL, HRAS, KRAS, LZTR1, MAP2A1, MAP2K2, NF1, NRAS, RAF1, RASA2, RIT1, RRAS, SHOC2, SOS1, SOS2,* and *SPRED1* genes have been uncovered as the molecular cause of NS or other closely related conditions, comprising NS with multiple lentigines (NSML, also known as LEOPARD syndrome; OMIM 151100), Noonan-like syndrome with loose anagen hair (NSLAH;

OMIN 607721), Costello syndrome (CS; OMIM 218040), cardiofaciocutaneous syndrome (CFC; OMIM 115150), neurofibromatosis type 1 (OMIM 162200), and Legius syndrome (OMIM 611431) [5]. Most of the genes associated with NS encoded proteins involved in RAS/MAPK signaling pathway. The mutations described in NS result in constitutive activation of producing proteins which disrupts RAS/MAPK signaling. Few mutations associated with NS are also described in genes which encoded proteins not involved in the RAS/MAPK signaling pathway [5]. The mechanism through which these mutations could lead to the signs and symptoms of NS has not been elucidated yet.

NS and these Noonan-like syndromes (NLS) are now designated as "RASopathies" because of clinical overlap and the similar molecular mechanisms disturbing the RAS/MAPK signaling pathway [6]. Despite the discovery of more than a dozen causative genes, molecular diagnosis remains a challenge in approximately 30% of patients with NS and NLS.

GROWTH PATTERN

Proportionate postnatal short stature is one of the cardinal signs of NS and is present in approximately 80% of individuals with this syndrome [7]. Birth weight and length are normal. However, height begins to drop down within the first year of life, and the mean height is below the lower limit of the standard population during childhood. The catch-up growth during puberty is attenuated in NS and patients reach an adult height below the normal range at the end of puberty [8].

The growth pattern of NS was first described before causative genes acknowledgement. Witt et al. evaluated 112 patients (64 males), in a cross-sectional mode, from birth to 60 years of age and obtained 173 measurements (1.5 observations/year per patient on average). The adult height reached at 18 years was 161 cm in men and 150.5 cm in women [9]. Later, Ranke et al. conducted a longitudinal study with 144 patients comprising 392 measurements in 89 males and 355 measures in 55 females from birth to age 19. Mean height in both sexes remained parallel to the third percentile of the reference curve for German population up to about 12 years in boys and 10 years in girls. Subsequently, mean height dropped below the normal range, reaching 162.5 and 152.7 cm in adult men and women, respectively. This decline was a result of the pubertal delay observed in these patients. In agreement with this observation, the bone age also presented a delay of

2 years regarding the chronological age. The growth curve proposed by Ranke et al. is used as the reference standard of NS to date [10].

In 2012, our group evaluated anthropometric measurements from birth to age 20 from 137 patients with NS and the related conditions (80 males), harboring a mutation in RAS/MAPK-related genes. One hundred twenty-five patients were evaluated in a longitudinal mode, resulting in 536 observations (average of 4.3 measurements per patient). Mean adult height was 157.4 cm (−2.4 SDS) and 148.4 cm (−2.2 SDS) for adult males and females, respectively, considering Brazilian healthy adult men and women [11]. Brazilian NS standards also described body mass index (BMI) in patients with NS and NLS. BMI in these patients was lower when compared to Brazilian children and adolescents from age 7 to 17 years. The authors argued that the inclusion of patients with only a confirmed molecular diagnosis reduced false diagnosis and allowed the presence of some individuals with subtle phenotype [8].

A Japanese growth chart was also designed for 308 individuals with a clinical and/or molecular diagnosis of NS. Genetic analysis was performed in 150 out of 308 patients and found causative mutations in 103 patients. Standards height, weight, and BMI charts were constructed with 3249 mixed longitudinal and cross-sectional measurements (1649 males). The mean adult height at the age of 20 years was 157.3 ± 7.4 cm for men and 146.8 ± 6.9 cm for women (-2.3 ± 1.3 and -2.1 ± 1.3 SDS for Japanese population) [12].

MECHANISMS OF GROWTH IMPAIRMENT

The physiopathological mechanism of growth retardation in NS remains unclear. The role of the GH-IGF-1 axis has been investigated by several researchers once GH is essential for normal postnatal growth. Low nocturnal levels and an unusual pulsatility of GH levels were first described in short-stature children with NS [13, 14]. Abnormal spontaneous GH secretion consistent with neurosecretory dysfunction has also been reported [15]. Stimulated and spontaneous GH levels are usually normal in patients with NS although a small number of patients may show a subnormal response [16, 17] depending on the considered cutoff of GH peak levels. Growth hormone deficiency (GHD) has been described in patients with NSLAH and mutations in the *SHOC2* gene [18].

Although NS and NSML are clinically overlapping disorders, some distinctive features are observed. Regarding prenatal growth, about one-third of patients with NSML present a birth weight within normal range or above. Short stature during childhood is less frequent in patients with NSML, being reported in only 25% of patients. Most of them reaches an adult height below the 25th centile. The *PTPN11* mutations related to NSML are grouped in exon 7, 12, and 13, and exhibit a reduced protein tyrosine phosphatase activity and are predicted to exert a dominant-negative effect in comparison with NS-*PTPN11* mutations [19].

GH exerts its action through binding to a specific receptor that phosphorylates several tyrosine residues located in the intracellular domain. SHP-2, encoded by *PTPN11* gene, participates in GH signaling dephosphorylating STAT5b. Physiologically, it results in downregulation of GH receptor activity [20]. Patients with *PTPN11* mutations present SHP-2 hyperactivation which could result in a postreceptor defect in GH action (Fig. 1). Several investigators have already reported that IGF-1 concentrations were low or at the lower limit of normality in patients with *PTPN11* mutations [21–23], while IGFBP-3 levels are normal [22, 24]. In animal models, low levels of IGF-1 were associated with growth retardation in an NS-mouse model with *Ptpn11* mutation because of ERK1/2 hyperactivation [25]. Taken together, normal or elevated GH levels along with low IGF-1 levels suggest a partial GH insensitivity in patients with NS and other RASopathies.

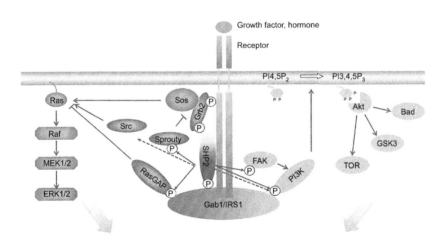

Fig. 1 Role of SHP2 in the activation of RAS/MAPK and PI3K/AKT signaling pathways downstream from tyrosine kinase receptors (TKR). *(From Tajan M, de Rocca Serra A, Valet P, Edouard T, Yart A. SHP2 sails from physiology to pathology. Eur J Med Genet 2015;58(10):509–25, Fig. 2, with permission.)*

Regardless of GH–IGF-1 axis, RAS/MAPK also exerts a direct effect on growth plate through a decrease in chondrocyte proliferation and terminal differentiation and cartilage matrix synthesis [26]. Gain-of-function mutations in *FGFR3* gene (OMIM*134934) lead to phosphorylation of the RAS/MAPK pathway increase and result in achondroplasia (ACH, OMIM*100800). Similarly, mutations in RAS/MAPK genes related to NS and NLS also increase ERK1/2 activation, and it could result in chondrocyte growth impairment. Moreover, induced germ-line inactivating mutations of *Ptpn11* gene in mice has revealed that osteoclastogenesis stimulated by M-CSF and RANKL was defective. Furthermore, heterozygous inactivating mutations in *PTPN11* gene were described in metachondromatosis (METCDS, OMIM#156250), a rare inherited disorder presenting with multiple exostoses, enchondromas, joint destruction and bony deformities [27]. Understanding the role of SHP2 and other proteins of RAS/MAPK signaling pathway in chondrocyte regulation will allow the development of new therapeutic approaches for patients with growth plate and skeletal malformations.

ROLE OF RAS/MAPK MUTATIONS IN GROWTH

The growth pattern was primarily described in the pregenomic era, and the discovery of the causative genes prompt investigators to seek genotype-phenotype correlations. In the literature, the frequency of short stature in NS is described as 73% in patients with *PTPN11,* 85% with *RAF1,* 84% in *KRAS,* and 35% in *SOS1* mutations. Patients with the *PTPN11* mutations related to NSML are less affected by short stature, in a frequency of 18% [28], probably because these mutations affect different residues of SHP2 resulting in decreased catalytic activity [29].

In a recent large French cohort of NS patients, the authors reported that patients with *PTPN11* and *RAF1* mutations had lower birth length and weight than the ones affected by *SOS1* and *KRAS* mutations. On the other hand, neonates with *KRAS* mutations had an increased frequency of macrosomia. Birth length was higher in patients with *SOS1* mutation and remained up to age 2 [28]. This observation agrees with a previous French study, which found a trend of lower birth length and higher frequency of small for gestational age (SGA) patients with *PTPN11* mutations [24], but it is in discordance with Brazilian cohort findings, which showed no differences between genotypes in relation to birth measurements [8].

A Japanese study found that NS individuals with *PTPN11* mutations might be 0.39 SDS shorter than those with *BRAF, KRAS, RAF1, RIT1, SHOC2,* and *SOS1* mutations [12]. Differently, Brazilian cohort disclosed that patients with *SHOC2* mutations, followed by *RAF1* mutations, were shorter than patients with mutations in *BRAF, KRAS, PTPN11,* and *SOS1.* Patients with *SOS1* and *BRAF* mutations were the tallest [8]. In the large French cohort, the adult height and the frequency of short stature were similar between genotypes [28].

Regarding BMI, patients with NS lack the gradual increase after BMI rebound age and remain thinner as adults [8, 12, 30], mostly males [12]. In contrast, Cessans et al. showed BMI within normal limits at the age of 2, 5, and 10. After puberty, it remained in the lower normal range [28]. Patients with *SHOC2* mutations were also thinner in the Brazilian cohort [8]. Interestingly, patients with *RAF1* and *BRAF* mutations presented the highest BMI SDS among other genotypes [8]. Insulin and leptin, two important hormones involved in satiety signals, also act through the RAS/MAPK pathway [31] and their action could be disrupted in RASopathies. Low BMI SDS seems to confer a protection phenotype against metabolic disease, but the mechanisms underlying energy control in NS are not entirely understood yet.

HUMAN RECOMBINANT GROWTH HORMONE THERAPY

Despite the unknown mechanism underlying short stature in NS, treatment with recombinant human growth hormone (rhGH) has been proposed to improve the adult height of NS subjects since the 1980s [32]. US Food and Drug Administration (FDA) has approved it since 2007 in a dose ranging from 33 to 66 μg/kg/day. In spite of FDA approval, the same has not been applied by the European Medicines Agency. Therefore, this opposing attitude may result in different strategies in the care of children with NS worldwide.

Data on GH treatment were recorded from observational studies and clinical studies/case reports. Observational studies were designed to document the efficacy and safety of GH therapy from enrolled patients with NS in large postmarketing studies [33–36]. The value of these surveys in comparison with standard randomized controlled trials as a source of reliable and representative data on NS population has been discussed recently [37]. Lack of information on molecular diagnosis, malformations related to NS, familial or sporadic cases, growth hormone-deficiency, and puberty, is a common disadvantage in these studies.

Additionally, several clinical studies/case reports have described growth velocity improvement in NS patients treated with rhGH during a follow-up period <5 years [13, 22, 34, 38–41] or concerning near-adult height [33, 35, 42] or adult height [18, 43, 44] (Table 1). Mean growth velocity increased from 4.6 ± 1.0 cm at baseline to 8.0 ± 1.4 cm, 6.2 ± 1.4 cm, and 6.2 ± 2.0 cm at the end of the first year, the second year, and third year of therapy, respectively (Table 2). However, none of these therapy studies in NS was a randomized controlled trial and has fulfilled the endocrine society criteria for high quality of evidence [45]. Consequently, the efficacy of rhGH therapy in short-stature children with NS has not been proven yet [32].

Separate groups have assessed the influence of *PTPN11* mutations on growth improvement. Previous studies have shown worsening of the short-term response in patients with mutations compared to patients without mutations in the *PTPN11* gene [21, 23, 24]. This observation has not been confirmed in other studies evaluating the response to rhGH therapy in patients with mutations in *PTPN11* [41, 44]. At the adult height, patients with *SHOC2* mutations presented a higher height gain than patients with *PTPN11* mutations (1.4 ± 1.2 vs 0.5 ± 0.7, considering national population standards) [18]. Randomized clinical trials are required to confirm the usefulness of rhGH treatment in patients with mutations related to RASopathies compared to untreated controls.

Pretreatment GH, IGF-I, and IGFBP-3 levels have no correlation with growth response to rhGH therapy [15], although mean IGF-I SDS has increased during the first year of rhGH treatment [44]. The hyperactivation of RAS/MAPK signaling pathway in animal models harboring *Ptpn11* mutation resulted in lower systemic IGF-1 production which was restored by a selective inhibitor of RAS/MAPK signaling [25]. Pharmacological inhibition of the RAS/MAPK pathway have improved growth in other mouse models with mutation related to RASopathies [2]. These studies highlighted the role of hyperactivation of RAS/MAPK signaling on different cellular types in patients with NS. Moreover, they may move therapeutic options toward specific inactivation of RAS/MAPK signaling in target cells which could represent a new field of research.

Table 1 Anthropometric data and outcomes of studies on adult or near-adult height[a] after recombinant human growth hormone treatment in patients with Noonan syndrome

Author and year	N (M:F)	Molecular diagnosis (N)	Familial cases	Target height SDS	rhGH dose (μg/kg/day)	Mean age at start	Pubertal at start (N)	Mean height SDS at start	Mean therapy duration (years)	Mean adult height (cm)	Mean AH or NAH (SDS)	Height gain after treatment (SDS)	Difference from AH to TH (SDS)
Kirk et al. (2001) [33]	10 (6:4)	N.A.	N.A.	−0.6 (±0.8)[b]	34	12.1 (±2.4)[b]	N.A.	−3.3 (±0.6)[b]	5.3 (±1.8)[b]	6M: 159.9 4F: 147.2	−2.3 (±0.5)	1.0 (±0.3)[b]	−2.8 (±1.8)[b]
Osio et al. (2005) [43]	18 (7:11)	N.A.	N.A.	N.A.	49.5	8.2 (±3.0)[b]	N.A.	−2.9 (±0.4)	7.5[c]	7M: 174.5 11F: 157.7	−1.2 (±1.0)	1.7 (±0.6)	N.A.
Noordam et al. (2008) [44]	29 (8:21)	24 (22 PTPN11)	9	−0.9	50	11.0 (±2.7)[c]	4	−2.8 (±0.7)[c]	6.4 (±2.3)[c]	21M: 171.3 8F: 157.3	−1.5 (±0.8)[c]	1.3 (±0.7)[c]	−2.2 (±0.9)[d]
Raaijmakers et al. (2008) [35]	24 (N.A.)	N.A.	N.A.	−0.4[c,e,f]	34	10.2[c,e]	N.A.	3.2[c,e]	7.6[c,e]	N.A.	N.A.	0.6[c,e]	N.A.
Romano et al. (2009) [42]	65 (30:35)	N.A.	N.A.	−0.3 (±0.7)[c]	47	11.6 (±3.0)[c]	12	−3.5 (±1.0)	5.6 (±2.6)[c]	N.A.	−2.1 (±1.0)	1.4 (±0.7)[c]	N.A.
Tamburrino et al. (2015) [18]	16 (8:8)	16 (10 PTPN11)	N.A.	−0.5 (±0.9)[c]	35	6.9 (±3.6)[c,f]	N.A.	−2.8 (±0.8)[c,f]	9.3 (±4.0)[c]	8M: 164.3 8F: 147.8	−2.2 (±0.7)[c]	N.A.	N.A.

[a] Near-adult height defined as growth velocity ≤2.5 cm/year or chronological age at least 14 years in females and 15 years in males.
[b] Data recalculated from the original article for Centers for Disease Control and Prevention (CDC) growth standards.
[c] Data reported in the original article and calculated to national standards.
[d] Data on sporadic cases.
[e] Median.
[f] Calculated for the whole cohort.

AH, adult height; NAH, near-adult height; TH, target height.

Table 2 Growth velocity (GV) at baseline, first year, second year, and third year of GH therapy in patients with Noonan syndrome

Author	Year	Molecular diagnosis (*PTPN11*)	N	Mean GV at baseline	Mean GV at first year	Mean GV at second year	Mean GV at third year
Cotterill et al. [22]	1996	N.A.	40	4.9 ± 0.2	8.5 ± 0.4		
De Schepper et al. [39]	1997	N.A.	23	4.5 ± 1.0	8.5 ± 1.5		
Kirk et al. [33]	2001	N.A.	35	4.8 ± 1.1	7.2 ± 1.7		
Macfarlane et al. [38]	2001	N.A.	23	4.4 ± 1.7	8.4 ± 1.7	6.2 ± 1.7	5.8 ± 1.7
Noordam et al. [15]	2001	N.A.	17	4.7 ± 1.0	8.7 (range: 6.1–11.7)		
Ogawa et al. [40]	2004	N.A.	14	4.8 ± 1.1	7.0 ± 1.2	5.5 ± 0.6	
Ferreira et al. [23]	2005	*PTPN11* (7/14)	14	4.1 ± 1.3	7.2 ± 1.7	6.3 ± 1.9	6.4 ± 2.7
Limal et al. [24]	2006	PTPN11 (15/25)	25	4.7 ± 1.1	7.9 ± 1.6	6.3 ± 1.5	
Jeong et al. [50]	2016	*PTPN11* (9/12)	15	4.6 ± 0.8	8.6 ± 1.5	6.8 ± 1.3	6.4 ± 1.5
Total			206	4.6 ± 1.0	8.0 ± 1.4	6.2 ± 1.4	6.2 ± 2.0

ADVERSE EFFECTS OF rhGH THERAPY

rhGH was approved for use in children with GH deficiency by the FDA in 1985. Since then, observational studies supported by manufacturers of rhGH have provided data on the safety of rhGH therapy. The cumulative safety data from these registries involve more than 120,000 children treated with rhGH and support a safety profile for approved indications. However, the long-term safety of rhGH therapy remains inconclusive and under investigation, specially concerning cancer and cerebrovascular diseases [46]. Once cancer and vasculogenesis could be linked to RAS/MAPK signaling, and GH/IGF-1 system, treatment with rhGH for short-stature children with NS should be carefully considered.

An important consideration when deciding on short-stature treatment in NS children regards the deleterious effects of rhGH on the development of myocardial hypertrophy in patients with cardiac defects or abnormal cardiac function. Studies explicitly addressing the effectiveness of rhGH therapy have not indicated any cause for concern [14, 22, 38]. However, in a large cohort of 252 patients, Romano et al. in 2009 reported three cardiac events during rhGH therapy: increased biventricular hypertrophy, hypertrophic cardiomyopathy, and supravalvular aortic stenosis [42]. Ferreira et al. also described a deterioration of cardiac function in the second year of treatment in a patient who had mild left ventricular hypertrophy before rhGH treatment. Although rhGH therapy had been interrupted, he underwent cardiac surgery 1 year later [23]. This patient was negative for *PTPN11* mutations at the time of the study but disclosed a *RAF1* mutation c.770C > T, Ser257Leu (rs80338796; *personal communication*). For these reasons, it is recommended basal and annual echocardiography in all NS patients on rhGH treatment.

Another point to consider is the small but well-established risk of malignancy in individuals with NS and the unknown effects of rhGH on this issue. It is important to note that *PTPN11* gene mutations, which are the most cause of NS, are at higher malignancy risk at baseline (see Chapter 9). The cumulative risk of developing a malignancy is 23% up to 55 years of age [47]. Somatic activating *RAS* mutations occur in approximately 30% of human cancers, and somatic *PTPN11* mutations are responsible for one-third of juvenile myelomonocytic leukemia (JMML) and, less frequently, other types of leukemia or solid tumors [48]. The most common cancers in NS are neuroblastoma, low-grade glioma, rhabdomyosarcoma, and acute leukemia [49]. For children with NS and NLS under rhGH treatment for short stature, it is advisable to monitor for cancer surveillance during therapy and after completion of rhGH therapy. The association of increased cancer risk should be included in the discussion with parents/patients/families at the time of initiating rhGH therapy.

CONCLUSIONS

Since the discovery of the molecular cause of NS, much knowledge has been accumulated on the role of the RAS/MAPK signaling pathway in the linear growth of the affected patients. At present, rhGH therapy presents good effectiveness and safety and is the treatment of choice for short stature, but other therapeutic options may be considered in the future.

REFERENCES

[1] Tartaglia M, Gelb BD. Noonan syndrome and related disorders: genetics and pathogenesis. Annu Rev Genomics Hum Genet 2005;6:45–68.
[2] Yart A, Edouard T. Noonan syndrome: an update on growth and development. Curr Opin Endocrinol Diabetes Obes 2018;25(1):67–73.
[3] van der Burgt I, Berends E, Lommen E, van Beersum S, Hamel B, Mariman E. Clinical and molecular studies in a large Dutch family with Noonan syndrome. Am J Med Genet 1994;53(2):187–91.
[4] Tartaglia M, Mehler EL, Goldberg R, Zampino G, Brunner HG, Kremer H, et al. Mutations in PTPN11, encoding the protein tyrosine phosphatase SHP-2, cause Noonan syndrome. Nat Genet 2001;29(4):465–8.
[5] Aoki Y, Niihori T, Inoue S, Matsubara Y. Recent advances in RASopathies. J Hum Genet 2016;61(1):33–9.
[6] Tidyman WE, Rauen KA. The RASopathies: developmental syndromes of Ras/MAPK pathway dysregulation. Curr Opin Genet Dev 2009;19(3):230–6.
[7] Tartaglia M, Gelb BD, Zenker M. Noonan syndrome and clinically related disorders. Best Pract Res Clin Endocrinol Metab 2011;25(1):161–79.
[8] Malaquias AC, Brasil AS, Pereira AC, Arnhold IJ, Mendonca BB, Bertola DR, et al. Growth standards of patients with Noonan and Noonan-like syndromes with mutations in the RAS/MAPK pathway. Am J Med Genet A 2012;158A(11):2700–6.
[9] Witt DR, Keena BA, Hall JG, Allanson JE. Growth curves for height in Noonan syndrome. Clin Genet 1986;30(3):150–3.
[10] Ranke MB, Heidemann P, Knupfer C, Enders H, Schmaltz AA, Bierich JR. Noonan syndrome: growth and clinical manifestations in 144 cases. Eur J Pediatr 1988;148(3):220–7.
[11] Silva DA, Pelegrini A, Petroski EL, Gaya AC. Comparison between the growth of Brazilian children and adolescents and the reference growth charts: data from a Brazilian project. J Pediatr 2010;86(2):115–20.
[12] Isojima T, Sakazume S, Hasegawa T, Ogata T, Nakanishi T, Nagai T, et al. Growth references for Japanese individuals with Noonan syndrome. Pediatr Res 2016;79(4):543–8.
[13] Ahmed ML, Foot AB, Edge JA, Lamkin VA, Savage MO, Dunger DB. Noonan's syndrome: abnormalities of the growth hormone/IGF-I axis and the response to treatment with human biosynthetic growth hormone. Acta Paediatr Scand 1991;80(4):446–50.

[14] Noordam C, Draaisma JM, van den Nieuwenhof J, van der Burgt I, Otten BJ, Daniels O. Effects of growth hormone treatment on left ventricular dimensions in children with Noonan's syndrome. Horm Res 2001;56(3–4):110–3.

[15] Noordam C, van der Burgt I, Sweep CG, Delemarre-van de Waal HA, Sengers RC, Otten BJ. Growth hormone (GH) secretion in children with Noonan syndrome: frequently abnormal without consequences for growth or response to GH treatment. Clin Endocrinol 2001;54(1):53–9.

[16] Westphal O. Growth hormone therapy in Noonan syndrome: growth response and characteristics. Horm Res 2009;72(Suppl. 2):41–5.

[17] Noonan JA. Noonan syndrome and related disorders: alterations in growth and puberty. Rev Endocr Metab Disord 2006;7(4):251–5.

[18] Tamburrino F, Gibertoni D, Rossi C, Scarano E, Perri A, Montanari F, et al. Response to long-term growth hormone therapy in patients affected by RASopathies and growth hormone deficiency: patterns of growth, puberty and final height data. Am J Med Genet A 2015;167A(11):2786–94.

[19] Sarkozy A, Digilio MC, Dallapiccola B. Leopard syndrome. Orphanet J Rare Dis 2008;3:13.

[20] Wit JM, de Luca F. Atypical defects resulting in growth hormone insensitivity. Growth Hormon IGF Res 2016;28:57–61.

[21] Binder G, Neuer K, Ranke MB, Wittekindt NE. PTPN11 mutations are associated with mild growth hormone resistance in individuals with Noonan syndrome. J Clin Endocrinol Metab 2005;90(9):5377–81.

[22] Cotterill AM, McKenna WJ, Brady AF, Sharland M, Elsawi M, Yamada M, et al. The short-term effects of growth hormone therapy on height velocity and cardiac ventricular wall thickness in children with Noonan's syndrome. J Clin Endocrinol Metab 1996;81(6):2291–7.

[23] Ferreira LV, Souza SA, Arnhold IJ, Mendonca BB, Jorge AA. PTPN11 (protein tyrosine phosphatase, nonreceptor type 11) mutations and response to growth hormone therapy in children with Noonan syndrome. J Clin Endocrinol Metab 2005;90(9):5156–60.

[24] Limal JM, Parfait B, Cabrol S, Bonnet D, Leheup B, Lyonnet S, et al. Noonan syndrome: relationships between genotype, growth, and growth factors. J Clin Endocrinol Metab 2006;91(1):300–6.

[25] De Rocca S-NA, Edouard T, Treguer K, Tajan M, Araki T, Dance M, et al. Noonan syndrome-causing SHP2 mutants inhibit insulin-like growth factor 1 release via growth hormone-induced ERK hyperactivation, which contributes to short stature. Proc Natl Acad Sci U S A 2012;109(11):4257–62.

[26] Vasques GA, Arnhold IJ, Jorge AA. Role of the natriuretic peptide system in normal growth and growth disorders. Horm Res Paediatr 2014;82(4):222–9.

[27] Yang W, Neel BG. From an orphan disease to a generalized molecular mechanism: PTPN11 loss-of-function mutations in the pathogenesis of metachondromatosis. Rare Dis 2013;1:e26657.

[28] Cessans C, Ehlinger V, Arnaud C, Yart A, Capri Y, Barat P, et al. Growth patterns of patients with Noonan syndrome: correlation with age and genotype. Eur J Endocrinol 2016;174(5):641–50.

[29] Kontaridis MI, Swanson KD, David FS, Barford D, Neel BG. PTPN11 (Shp2) mutations in LEOPARD syndrome have dominant negative, not activating, effects. J Biol Chem 2006;281(10):6785–92.

[30] Bertola DR, Yamamoto GL, Almeida TF, Buscarilli M, Jorge AA, Malaquias AC, et al. Further evidence of the importance of RIT1 in Noonan syndrome. Am J Med Genet A 2014;164A(11):2952–7.

[31] Schwartz MW, Seeley RJ. Seminars in medicine of the Beth Israel Deaconess Medical Center. Neuroendocrine responses to starvation and weight loss. N Engl J Med 1997;336(25):1802–11.

[32] Giacomozzi C, Deodati A, Shaikh MG, Ahmed SF, Cianfarani S. The impact of growth hormone therapy on adult height in Noonan syndrome: a systematic review. Horm Res Paediatr 2015;83(3):167–76.

[33] Kirk JM, Betts PR, Butler GE, Donaldson MD, Dunger DB, Johnston DI, et al. Short stature in Noonan syndrome: response to growth hormone therapy. Arch Dis Child 2001;84(5):440–3.

[34] Romano AA, Blethen SL, Dana K, Noto RA. Growth hormone treatment in Noonan syndrome: the National Cooperative Growth Study experience. J Pediatr 1996;128(5 Pt 2):S18–21.

[35] Raaijmakers R, Noordam C, Karagiannis G, Gregory JW, Hertel NT, Sipila I, et al. Response to growth hormone treatment and final height in Noonan syndrome in a large cohort of patients in the KIGS database. J Pediatr Endocrinol Metab 2008;21 (3):267–73.

[36] Lee PA, Ross J, Germak JA, Gut R. Effect of 4 years of growth hormone therapy in children with Noonan syndrome in the American Norditropin studies: web-enabled research (ANSWER) program(R) registry. Int J Pediatr Endocrinol 2012;2012(1):15.

[37] Ranke MB. Noonan syndrome: growth to growth hormone—the experience of observational studies. Horm Res 2009;72(Suppl. 2):36–40.

[38] MacFarlane CE, Brown DC, Johnston LB, Patton MA, Dunger DB, Savage MO, et al. Growth hormone therapy and growth in children with Noonan's syndrome: results of 3 years' follow-up. J Clin Endocrinol Metab 2001;86(5):1953–6.

[39] De Schepper J, Otten BJ, Francois I, Bourguignon JP, Craen M, Van der Burgt I, et al. Growth hormone therapy in pre-pubertal children with Noonan syndrome: first year growth response and comparison with turner syndrome. Acta Paediatr 1997;86 (9):943–6.

[40] Ogawa M, Moriya N, Ikeda H, Tanae A, Tanaka T, Ohyama K, et al. Clinical evaluation of recombinant human growth hormone in Noonan syndrome. Endocr J 2004;51 (1):61–8.

[41] Şıklar Z, Genens M, Poyrazoğlu Ş, Baş F, Darendeliler F, Bundak R, et al. The growth characteristics of patients with Noonan syndrome: results of three years of growth hormone treatment: a nationwide multicenter study. J Clin Res Pediatr Endocrinol 2016;8 (3):305–12.

[42] Romano AA, Dana K, Bakker B, Davis DA, Hunold JJ, Jacobs J, et al. Growth response, near-adult height, and patterns of growth and puberty in patients with Noonan syndrome treated with growth hormone. J Clin Endocrinol Metab 2009;94(7):2338–44.

[43] Osio D, Dahlgren J, Wikland KA, Westphal O. Improved final height with long-term growth hormone treatment in Noonan syndrome. Acta Paediatr 2005;94(9):1232–7.

[44] Noordam C, Peer PG, Francois I, De Schepper J, van den Burgt I, Otten BJ. Long-term GH treatment improves adult height in children with Noonan syndrome with and without mutations in protein tyrosine phosphatase, non-receptor-type 11. Eur J Endocrinol 2008;159(3):203–8.

[45] Swiglo BA, Murad MH, Schünemann HJ, Kunz R, Vigersky RA, Guyatt GH, et al. A case for clarity, consistency, and helpfulness: state-of-the-art clinical practice guidelines in endocrinology using the grading of recommendations, assessment, development, and evaluation system. J Clin Endocrinol Metab 2008;93(3):666–73.

[46] Sävendahl L, Pournara E, Pedersen BT, Blankenstein O. Is safety of childhood growth hormone therapy related to dose? Data from a large observational study. Eur J Endocrinol 2016;174(5):681–91.

[47] Jongmans MC, van der Burgt I, Hoogerbrugge PM, Noordam K, Yntema HG, Nillesen WM, et al. Cancer risk in patients with Noonan syndrome carrying a PTPN11 mutation. Eur J Hum Genet 2011;19(8):870–4.

[48] Schubbert S, Shannon K, Bollag G. Hyperactive Ras in developmental disorders and cancer. Nat Rev Cancer 2007;7(4):295–308.

[49] Noonan JA, Kappelgaard AM. The efficacy and safety of growth hormone therapy in children with Noonan syndrome: a review of the evidence. Horm Res Paediatr 2015;83 (3):157–66.

[50] Jeong I, Kang E, Cho JH, Kim GH, Lee BH, Choi JH, et al. Long-term efficacy of recombinant human growth hormone therapy in short-statured patients with Noonan syndrome. Ann Pediatr Endocrinol Metab 2016;21(1):26–30.

CHAPTER 3

Cardiac Manifestations in Noonan Syndrome: Effects of Growth Hormone Therapy

Ronak J. Naik
Division of Cardiology, Department of Pediatrics, Le Bonheur Children's Hospital, University of Tennessee Health Science Center, Memphis, TN, United States

Abstract

Noonan syndrome (NS) is an autosomal dominant disorder with prevalence of 1:1000 to 1:2500. Cardiac defects are present in up to 70%–80% of patients, pulmonary valve stenosis (PS) being the most common in about 50% followed by atrial septal defect (ASD) in ~20% and then hypertrophic cardiomyopathy (HCM) in ~15%. PTPN11 has predilection toward PS and ASD but rarely with HCM or coarctation of aorta. HCM is more common in NS compared to general population. RAF1, BRAF1, RIT1 mutations have HCM as major feature in NS. PS in majority remains mild without progression and likely from dysplastic valve. At least 1/3rd patients respond well to balloon angioplasty requiring reintervention in remaining 2/3rd patients. In more than half of the patients, HCM is mild with rare progression and favorable prognosis. Severe HCM diagnosed before 1 year of age has higher mortality and poor prognosis. The long-term data on survival in NS patients with HCM is acceptable; however, long-term studies are needed to answer this question. ASDs are generally treated in line with the standard methodologies. Various other cardiac defects like ventricular septal defects, atrioventricular septal defect, aortic and mitral valve problems, branch pulmonary artery stenoses, coarctation of aorta, and aortic root dilation have also been observed. Growth hormone therapy is rarely associated with adverse cardiac events making it largely a safe therapy.

Keywords: Noonan syndrome, Cardiac manifestations, Growth hormone

Abbreviations

ASD	atrial septal defect
GH	growth hormone
HCM	hypertrophic cardiomyopathy
LVH	left ventricular hypertrophy
LVOT	left ventricular outflow tract
MAPK	mitogen activated protein kinase
NS	Noonan syndrome
PS	pulmonary valve stenosis
VSD	ventricular septal defect

Noonan Syndrome
https://doi.org/10.1016/B978-0-12-815348-2.00002-5

INTRODUCTION

Noonan syndrome (NS) is an autosomal dominant disorder with complete penetrance but variable expression. Its prevalence is estimated at 1 in 1000 to 1 in 2500 [1, 2]. Dr. Jacqueline Noonan first recognized it in 1963 as a syndrome with typical facial features, short stature, and congenital heart disease [3]. Since its first recognition, several phenotypes closely related to NS have been described currently known as "Noonan syndrome spectrum" or RASopathies. It includes Noonan syndrome (NS), Noonan syndrome with multiple lentigines (NSML; previously known as LEOPARD syndrome), Costello syndrome, Cardiofaciocutaneous (CFC) syndrome, neurofibromatosis type I (NF-1), and Legius syndrome. Congenital heart disease has been a major feature of NS. Over the years, types and characteristics of congenital heart disease are well understood. Management of these defects has evolved to change long-term outcome. With the advent of growth hormone (GH) therapy, increased growth velocity and adult height can be achieved. Effect of GH therapy on cardiac issues is being studied. For the review of literature in this chapter, we will focus on cardiac manifestations in Noonan syndrome from among the various RASopathies.

GENETICS

Genetic mutations are present in about 61% of the patients [4]. The first gene identified was *PTPN11* which encodes the protein SHP2 on region of chromosome 12q24.1 linked to NS [5]. RAS/mitogen-activated protein kinase (MAPK) pathway is an important signal transduction pathway leading to cell proliferation and differentiation. Till date, 12 genes have been identified in the RAS-MAPK pathway linked to NS. Fig. 1 shows some of the gene mutations in RAS-MAPK pathway resulting in Noonan syndrome spectrum disorders [6]. A new LZTR1 gene, unrelated to RAS-MAPK pathway, has been found to be associated with NS [7]. Recently, another novel de novo missense mutation in protein phosphatase 1 catalytic subunit beta (PPP1CB) is shown to have phenotypic features closely mimicking NS with loose anagen hair [8]. Table 1 presents gene mutations, type of mutations, prevalence, and most common cardiac defects [9].

CARDIAC MANIFESTATIONS

Cardiac abnormality is one of the most common feature of NS being present in more than 80% [4]. NS is the second most common syndromic causes of congenital heart defects [10]. Table 2 presents comparison of prevalence from some of the published NS cohorts.

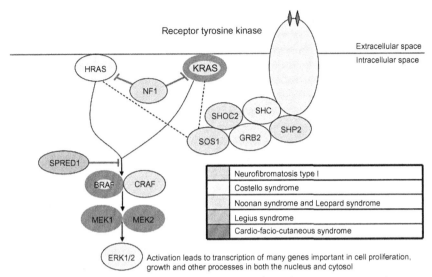

Fig. 1 The RAS-MAPK pathway and disorders resulting from mutations in its gene. SHP-2 protein is product of PTPN11 gene. *(With permission from Burkitt Wright E, Kerr B. RAS-MAPK pathway disorders: important causes of congenital heart disease, feeding difficulties, developmental delay and short stature. Arch Dis Child 2010;95:724–30).*

Most common congenital heart defect is pulmonary valve stenosis (PS) with dysplastic pulmonary valve, found in ~50% of cases. Traditionally secundum atrial septal defect (ASD) was thought to be around 6%–10%; however, based on cumulative cohort in Table 2 the occurrence is around ~20% making it the second most common heart defect in NS. Hypertrophic cardiomyopathy (HCM) is found in ~15% of NS cases. Ventricular septal defect (VSD) is the next most common after HCM followed by patent ductus arteriosus, mitral valve disorders, branch pulmonary artery stenoses, and aortic valve disorders in decreasing order. Other less common structural heart defects that occur in NS are partial atrioventricular septal defect, tetralogy of Fallot, patent ductus arteriosus, coarctation of aorta, aortic root dilation, and subaortic stenosis [19,20]. Rarely pulmonary hypertension, Ebstein's anomaly, pulmonary atresia, coronary artery anomalies, dilated cardiomyopathy can also be present. Table 3 presents the spectrum of different cardiac defects reported in NS.

Abnormal electrocardiographic findings are noted in up to 50% of patients with NS regardless of presence of underlying cardiovascular abnormality [21]. These findings include left axis deviation, giant Q wave, and abnormal R/S ratio.

Prevalence of congenital heart disease also varies with each gene mutations.

Table 1 Noonan syndrome: gene mutations, prevalence, and types of cardiac defects

Mutation in gene	Proportion of NS attributed to gene mutation (%)	Type of mutation	Prevalence of cardiac defects (%)	Most common type of cardiac defect
RAF1	5–15	Gain of function	80–95	HCM
PTPN11	50	Mis-sense, gain of function	74–80	PS and ASD
SOS1	10–13	Mis-sense	80	Septal defects, ASD; second most common mutation for PS
KRAS	<5	Gain of function	65–85	Similar to PTPN11 but mild
RIT1	5	Mis-sense	70–75	HCM
LZTR1 and SOS2	3	Mis-sense, gain of function	NK	PS, ASD, HCM, mitral valve disorders, coarctation
NRAS	<2	Gain of function	NK	NK
BRAF	<2	Gain of function	NK	HCM
MAP2K1 or MAP2K2	<2	Mis-sense	NK	HCM
SHOC2	<1	Missense	NK	MV dysplasia, ASD
PPP1CB	<1	Missense	NK	Congenital Heart Disease

ASD, atrial septal defect; *HCM*, hypertrophic cardiomyopathy; *MV*, mitral valve; *NK*, not known; *PS*, pulmonary valve stenosis.
Adapted and modified from Allanson JE, Roberts AE, Noonan syndrome. © University of Washington 1993–2017. GeneReviews® is a registered trademark of the University of Washington, Seattle. The content is used with permission. All rights reserved.

Table 2 Prevalence of cardiac defects in patients with NS in selective published large cohorts

	Jhang et al. [11]	Colquitt et al. [12]	Prendiville et al. [13]	Sznajer et al. [14]	Jongmans et al. [15]	Zenker et al. [16]	Sarkozy et al. [17]	Tartaglia et al. [18]	Cumulative occurrence (number)	Cumulative occurrence (%) of cardiac defect per total NS patients	Cumulative occurrence (%) of cardiac defect per number of NS patients with cardiac defects
Cohort sample size	119	113	293	272	103	57	81	119	1157	100%	100%
Patients with cardiac defect	92	102	237	200	75	NA	74	100	880	76.06	100%
Pulmonary valve stenosis	51	75	166	115	44	42	30	66	589	50.91	66.93
Atrial septal defects	39	5	94	48	21	10	6	17	240	20.74	27.27
Hypertrophic cardiomyopathy	22	16	47	48	4	9	7	20	173	14.95	19.66
Atrioventricular septal defect	NA	NA	NA	5	NA	NA	9	NA	14	NP	NP
Coarctation of aorta	4	NA	7	11	NA	NA	4	NA	26	NP	NP
Ventricular septal defects	15	3	35	30	NA	8	3	NA	94	NP	NP
Aortic valve problem	NA	1	19	10	NA	NA	NA	NA	30	NP	NP
Mitral valve problem	NA	2	17	17	NA	NA	3	NA	39	NP	NP

Continued

Table 2 Prevalence of cardiac defects in patients with NS in selective published large cohorts—cont'd

	Jhang et al.	Colquitt et al.	Prendiville et al.	Sznajer et al.	Jongmans et al.	Zenker et al.	Sarkozy et al.	Tartaglia et al.	Cumulative occurrence (number)	Cumulative occurrence (%) of cardiac defect per total NS patients	Cumulative occurrence (%) of cardiac defect per number of NS patients with cardiac defects
Branch pulmonary artery stenosis	4	NA	NA	33	NA	NA	NA	NA	37	NP	NP
Tetralogy of Fallot	5	2	5	NA	NA	NA	NA	NA	12	NP	NP
Patent ductus arteriosus	21	3	26	NA	NA	NA	NA	NA	50	NP	NP
Subaortic stenosis	NA	2	NA	NA	NA	NA	NA	NA	2	NP	NP
Aortic root dilation	NA	NA	15	NA	NA	NA	NA	NA	15	NP	NP

NA, not available; *NP*, not possible.

Table 3 Spectrum of heart defects in Noonan syndrome

More common	Less common	Rare
Pulmonary valve stenosis	Ventricular septal defect	Aortic root dilation
Secundum ASD	Patent ductus arteriosus	Pulmonary atresia
Hypertrophic cardiomyopathy	Mitral valve abnormality	Subaortic stenosis
	Branch pulmonary artery stenosis	Ebstein's anomaly
	Aortic valve disorder	Dilated cardiomyopathy
	Coarctation of aorta	Coronary artery abnormalities
	Tetralogy of Fallot	

PTPN11 encoded protein SHP2 plays important role in semilunar valvulogenesis [22]. Missense or gain-of-function mutation in PTPN11 leading to prolonged activation of the protein accounts for 50% of NS cases [18,23]. Pulmonary valve stenosis and/or atrial septal defects are the most common cardiac anomalies in individuals with PTPN11 whereas coarctation of aorta and HCM are rare [5, 18]. Deletion of PTPN11 exon 2 results in dysplastic pulmonary valve.

With RAF1 gain-of-function mutation—HCM is present in 95% of cases in contrast to 20%–30% in overall NS indicating that increase in RAS signaling from gain-of-function mutation can lead to cardiomyocyte hypertrophy. Second most common mutation associated with HCM in NS is RIT1 with prevalence of 70%–75% [24,25]. BRAF, MAP2K1 mutations have HCM as more common phenotype. SOS1 mis-sense mutation is more associated with septal defects specifically atrial septal defects [26]. KRAS mutation has milder gain-of-function effect which is associated with cardiac anomalies in 85% of cases [27]. Mitral valve dysplasia and septal defects are more common in SHOC2 mutation [28]. Phenotypic variability has been observed with different mutations of same gene LZTR1 which emphasizes the importance of detail cardiac evaluation in any child with NS or NS-like features [7]. PPP1CB is a major serine/threonine specific protein phosphatase involved in the development of angiogenesis and endothelial migration; and in mice model cardiac-specific deletion of PPP1CB resulted in concentric remodeling of the heart, interstitial fibrosis, and contractile dysfunction [29,30].

PULMONARY VALVE STENOSIS

Dysplastic pulmonary valve is found in 25%–35% of pulmonary valve stenosis patients in NS [14]. Such valves have hypoplastic annulus, thickened cusps, and little fusion. Poststenotic dilation is generally less common in dysplastic pulmonary valve. Children usually present early with a heart murmur. Echocardiogram is the tool of choice for diagnosis. Fig. 2 demonstrates parasternal short axis view of pulmonary valve. Echocardiogram provides information about the size of pulmonary valve, leaflet motion, degree of stenosis, presence/absence of poststenotic dilation, degree of right ventricular hypertrophy, and right ventricular function. Mild PS can be managed conservatively. For moderate or severe PS or in symptomatic patient, percutaneous balloon angioplasty is usually performed. In the presence of dysplastic valve percutaneous balloon valvuloplasty has higher reintervention rate. Fig. 3 demonstrates pulmonary valve appearance on cardiac catheterization angiography and during balloon angioplasty. With severe pulmonary valve dysplasia surgical valvotomy and/or supravalvar patch augmentation may be required. If resultant pulmonary valve insufficiency becomes severe then surgical pulmonary valve placement may become necessary later in life.

Literature is largely lacking for long-term follow-up of NS patients' cardiac defects. Two recent studies have documented long-term outcomes for

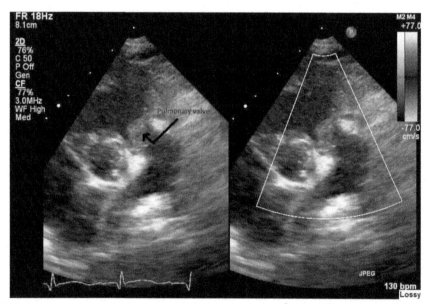

Fig. 2 Echocardiogram of pulmonary valve in NS. *Arrow* depicts thick pulmonary valve.

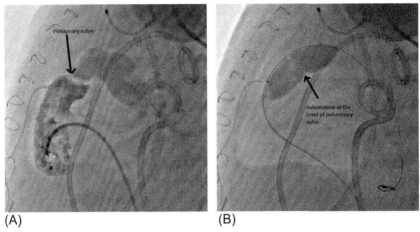

Fig. 3 Pulmonary valve on cardiac catheterization (A) At baseline a thick pulmonary valve appears as a white structure during contrast injection, (B) During balloon angioplasty. Waist on the balloon indicates level of pulmonary valve.

cardiac sequelae of NS. Colquitt el al had 66% ($n = 75$) of NS patients with PS out of 113 total [12]. More than half, 57% ($n = 43$) had mild PS. Patients with mild PS did not require intervention like in patients without NS. Notably, only two patients out of 43 mild PS patients had dysplastic pulmonary valve. Average age of diagnosis for mild or moderate PS in this cohort was around ~2.5 years. Out of seven (9%) patients with moderate PS only three required intervention on average 12.5 years after the diagnosis. Severe PS was diagnosed later at an average age of 6.2 years in 33% ($n = 25$) of patients. Out of these 25, 3 had balloon valvuloplasty while the rest requiring surgical intervention. Rate of reintervention had not been mentioned in this study. Another large cohort published by Prendiville et al. had 57% ($n = 166$) patients with PS out of 293 patients of NS [13]. Out of all patients with PS again, more than half—53% ($n = 88$)—patients did not require intervention. Percutaneous balloon valvuloplasty was required in 25% ($n = 43$) patients out of which 65% (21 surgery and 7 repeat balloon valvuloplasty) required reintervention which is in contrast to 10% quoted in earlier studies [31,32]. Out of 58 patients requiring surgery (initial approach and failed balloon valvuloplasty) 24% ($n = 14$) had transannular patch, 64% ($n = 37$) pulmonary valvotomy, and 12% ($n = 7$) had combination of procedures. While only 4% ($n = 7$) required pulmonary valve replacement, author concluded this as an underestimation due to lower median age of cohort of 14 years.

HYPERTROPHIC CARDIOMYOPATHY

HCM is a disease state characterized by unexplained left ventricular hypertrophy (LVH) associated with nondilated ventricular chambers in the absence of another cardiac or systemic disease being entirely responsible for the magnitude of hypertrophy evident in a given patient. Clinically, HCM is usually recognized by maximal LV wall thickness more than or equal to 15 mm, with wall thickness of 13–14 mm considered borderline, particularly in the presence of other compelling information (e.g., family history of HCM). In children, increased LV wall thickness in HCM is defined as wall thickness more than or equal to 2 SD (SD = standard deviation) above the mean (Z score $\geq$2) for age, sex, or body size.

Its prevalence in general population is 0.2% (1:500); however, in NS it is about 15%. It has predilection toward certain mutations as noted in Table 1. More than half of the times it is present in conjunction with other cardiac defects. HCM can be asymmetrical septal hypetrophy, apical, lateral wall, or concentric. No studies till date have described morphologic types of HCM for different NS mutations. Majority of children are asymptomatic from mild HCM. More than 50% of patients with NS and HCM are diagnosed by age of 6 months. Infants presenting before 6 months of age with congestive heart failure have the worst prognosis [33,34]. In older patients, chest pain, syncope, palpitations, dizziness, or dyspnea can be present. Positive family history is a risk factor for developing similar phenotype. In significant hypertrophy, electrocardiogram (EKG) may demonstrate voltage criteria for hypertrophy, deep and narrow Q waves, and/or T wave inversions. Echocardiography remains the mainstay for diagnosis. It helps in localizing the hypertrophy, quantifying the degree of left ventricular outflow tract (LVOT) obstruction, mitral valve involvement, left ventricular systolic and diastolic function, and so on. Fig. 4 shows myocardial hypertrophy in two different patients. Cardiac magnetic resonance imaging can be helpful in looking for fibrosis.

Course of HCM varies significantly from complete resolution to severe left ventricular obstruction. For symptomatic patients, traditional therapies include beta-blockers or calcium channel blocker. Ionotropic agents and vasodilators are contraindicated in obstructive HCM. Diuretics can be used very cautiously. Antiarrhythmics should be considered for intractable arrhythmias. For chronic arrhythmias, anticoagulation may also be necessary. Surgical myomectomy is reserved for the patients with LVOT pressure gradient of >50 mmHg and failed medical management. Alcohol septal

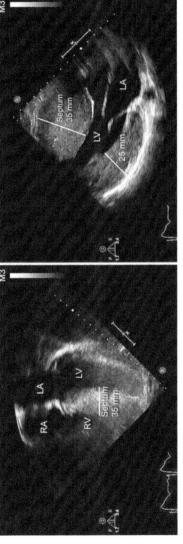

Fig. 4 Echocardiograms of hypertrophic cardiomyopathy involving left ventricle.

ablation, dual chamber pacemaker, or mitral valve replacement is very rarely required in children. Overall prognosis for mild HCM in NS is good. Studies comparing long-term HCM outcomes in NS vs nonsyndromic patients have demonstrated varying results. Colquitt et al. had 14% ($n = 16$) HCM occurrence in cohort of 113 out of which 9 (56%) were mild [12]. Only two patients from mild HCM progressed to moderate HCM. Among 7 (44%) of severe HCM one died postmyectomy at 6 months of age and another at 10 years of age. One important observation authors made was that of unlikelihood of HCM progression or new onset HCM beyond infancy and early childhood. Prendiville et al. looked at their cohort of 293 NS patients in more detail [13]. From 47 (16%) HCM patients, more than half were diagnosed in first year of life. Authors suggested this may be due to screening once NS is diagnosed/suspected. NS mutation was identified in 44% ($n = 21$) patients with HCM. In more than 70% of patients HCM was associated with other cardiac defects. Severe HCM was present in 18 (38%) patients out of which 5 requiring intervention. Seven HCM patients died of which four were diagnosed before 1 year of age conferring 15% mortality to <1 year group. Seventeen percent ($n = 8$) patients have spontaneous regression from which two had severe HCM. Authors predicted >80% survival of NS patients with HCM at 25 years of age with still 10% at risk.

ATRIAL SEPTAL DEFECTS

Atrial septal defects can be of secundum type or primum type. Presentation can be delayed for up to 1–2 years in isolated small–moderate size defects. Majority of the time presence of typical facial features of NS would warrant thorough testing which includes echocardiogram making ASDs in NS getting diagnosed early in the course. Fig. 5 demonstrates an echocardiographic image of secundum ASD. Small defects can be managed conservatively as an outpatient. Spontaneous closure rate is very high in small ASDs during the first 4 years of life. Moderate or large defects may lead to right atrial and right ventricular enlargement. Moderate defects, if tolerated well, can be closed around 2–3 years with device in cardiac catheterization lab (Fig. 6). Large defects or symptomatic patient not suitable for device closure may require surgical patch closure of the defect. Long-term prognosis of repaired ASDs has remained excellent with minimal complications. ASDs in NS have similar course-like patients without NS.

Other cardiac defects are managed in standard ways.

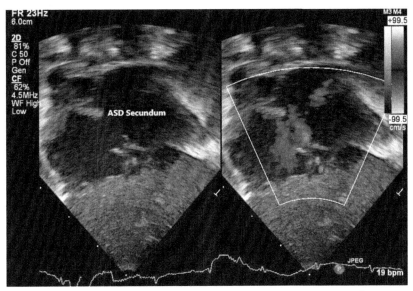

Fig. 5 Echocardiogram of the secundum ASD. *Left frame* shows large secundum ASD on 2-dimentional image. *Right frame* shows color across the ASD indicating left to right flow.

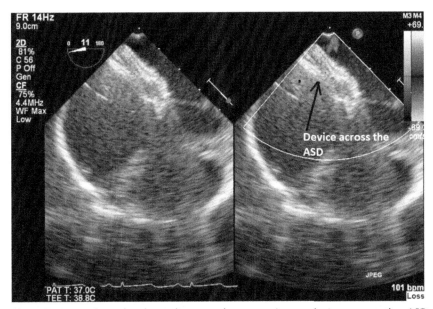

Fig. 6 Transesophageal echocardiogram demonstrating a device across the ASD closing the defect.

EFFECT OF GROWTH HORMONE THERAPY

Short stature is one of the more common features of NS occurring in 50%–70% of patients [2, 35]. Variation of prevalence among mutations is noted with PTPN11 being higher and SOS1 being lower. Growth hormone (GH) therapy has improved growth velocity in NS patients. Anabolic effect of growth hormone may affect cardiomyocyte. Long-term effects of GH excess from intrinsic endocrine problems have been studied in acromegaly. In those patients, cardiac hypertrophy has been observed after prolonged exposure to increased GH level. Peripheral and pulmonary vasodilatory effects are predominant in short-term usage [36]. Several studies have examined the effect of GH on cardiac function in NS. Cotterill et al. in 1996 performed prospective case-control study [37]. Twenty-seven out of 30 children with NS completed GH treatment for 12 months. Comparing to 10 controls with NS, no increase in mean maximal LV wall thickness noted. The National Cooperative Growth Study (NCGS) examined response to 4 years of GH therapy in 150 children with NS and found no adverse cardiac events [38]. In 2009 same author published another study of 370 NS children from NCGS cohort treated with GH for a mean of 5.6 years [39]. Cardiac defects were present in 46% of the cohort. Only three adverse cardiac events (biventricular hypertrophy, HCM, and supravalvar aortic stenosis) reported which were considered to be comorbidities of NS. Noordam et al. divided 27 children in two groups: First group receiving high dose GH therapy in year 1 and 2; Second group receiving high dose GH therapy in year 2 and 3 [40]. The groups were followed for total of 4 years. Authors reported no significant differences in LV dimensions at baseline and after GH therapy in two groups after 4 years follow-up. Interesting fact was that there was only one patient with HCM in the group. Another study by same author on 27 children with NS receiving GH therapy demonstrated two children progressing from mild PS, one of them requiring balloon angioplasty [41]. Results of GH therapy in 429 children with NS were published in 2007 from Pfizer International Growth Database (KIGS) [42]. Cardiac events were reported in seven children. Minimum treatment duration was 2 years before cardiac side effects were noted. Cardiomyopathy resulting in heart transplant in one patient and severe LV hypertrophy in another patient reported. Three children developed arrhythmias, one angina and one had cyanotic episode. In one recent study Zavras et al. compared GH therapy efficacy in 5 NS GH deficient and 5 idiopathic GH deficient children for 5 years [43]. No severe cardiac adverse events are reported.

Thus there is a growing evidence that GH therapy is safer from cardiac perspective in children with NS though there remain rare adverse events. In this regard continuous cardiac follow-up becomes necessary.

In 2010 management guidelines for Noonan syndrome were published. Recommendations for management of cardiovascular issues based on this guideline are as follows [4]:

1. All individuals should undergo a cardiac evaluation by a cardiologist at the time of diagnosis, including an electrocardiogram and echocardiogram.

2. Those found to have cardiac problems should have regular follow-up at intervals determined by the cardiologist; cardiac care should be individualized according to the specific disorder(s) present.

3. Some will require treatment such as balloon valvuloplasty or surgery; long-term reevaluation of these patients after treatment is essential (specifically, after successful cardiac surgery, cardiac care should not be discontinued).

4. Individuals without heart disease on their initial evaluation should have cardiac reevaluation every 5 year.

5. Adults should not discontinue periodic cardiac evaluations even if their evaluations in childhood or adolescence were normal; unexpected cardiac findings can occur at any point in time.

In summary, Noonan syndrome now has more defined genetic mutations linked with different cardiac defects. Cardiac defects are most consistent feature of NS in children although can also develop in adult life. PTPN11 mutation is associated with PS and ASD while rarely with coarctation of aorta and HCM. HCM on the contrary is a common feature of RAF1, BRAF, and RIT1 mutations. ASD appears to be the second most common cardiac defect after PS in NS population. Dysplastic pulmonary valve is more common cause of PS with more than half being in mild category. Mild PS does not progress in majority. Almost 2/3 patients would require reintervention postballoon valvuloplasty in moderate or severe PS. HCM in majority remains mild with good long-term prognosis. However, severe HCM diagnosed <6 months of life or with cardiac failure has worst prognosis. Current survival of HCM in NS is likely greater than 80% at 25 years of age. Further long-term studies to learn more about frequency of pulmonary valve placement, to know morphology of HCM, to know rate of progression and long-term outcome of HCM and survival outcomes are needed. GH therapy is largely safe with rare cardiac events. Thus routine lifelong cardiac follow-up becomes necessary.

CONFLICT OF INTEREST

There are no conflict of interest for the author of this manuscript.

REFERENCES

[1] Nora JJ, Nora AH, Sinha AK, Spangler RD, Lubs HA. The Ullrich-Noonan syndrome (Turner phenotype). Am J Dis Child 1974;127:48–55.

[2] Mendez HM, Opitz JM. Noonan syndrome: a review. Am J Med Genet 1985;21:493–506.

[3] Noonan JA, Ehmke DA. Associated noncardiac malformations in children with congenital heart disease. J Pediatr 1963;31:150–3.

[4] Romano AA, Allanson JE, Dahlgren J, Gelb BD, Hall B, Pierpont ME, Roberts AE, Robinson W, Takemoto CM, Noonan JA. Noonan syndrome: clinical features, diagnosis, and management guidelines. Pediatrics 2010;126:746–59.

[5] Tartaglia M, Mehler EL, Goldberg R, Zampino G, Brunner HG, Kremer H, van der Burgt I, Crosby AH, Ion A, Jeffery S, Kalidas K, Patton MA, Kucherlapti RS, Gelb BD. Mutations in PTPN11, encoding the protein tyrosine phosphatase SHP-2, cause Noonan syndrome. Nat Genet 2001;29:465–8.

[6] Burkitt Wright EMM, Kerr B. RAS-MAPK pathway disorders: important causes of congenital heart disease, feeding difficulties, developmental delay and short stature. Arch Dis Child 2010;95:724–30.

[7] Yamamoto GL, Aguena M, Gos M, Hung C, Pilch J, Fahiminiya S, Abramowics A, Cristian I, Buscarilli M, Naslavsky MS, Malaquias AC, Zatz M, Bodamer O, Majewski J, Jorge AAL, Pereira AC, Kim CA, Passos-Bueno MR, Bertola DR. Rare variants in SOS2 and LZTR1 are associated with Noonan syndrome. J Med Genet 2015;52(6):413–21.

[8] Gripp KW, Aldinger KA, Bennett JT, Baker L, Tusi J, Powell-Hamilton N, Stabley D, Sol-Church K, Timms AE, Dobyns WB. A novel rasopathy caused by recurrent de novo missense mutations in PPP1CB closely resembles Noonan syndrome wit loose anagen hair. Am J Med Genet A 2016;170(9):2237–47.

[9] Allanson JE, Roberts AE. Noonan syndrome. In: Adam MP, Ardinger HH, Pagon RA, et al., GeneReviews®. Seattle, WA: University of Washington; 1993–2018 Available from: https://www.ncbi.nlm.nih.gov/books/NBK1124/.

[10] Marino B, Digilio MC, Toscano A, Giannotti A, Dallapiccola B. Congenital heart diseases in children with Noonan syndrome: an expanded cardiac spectrum with high prevalence of atrioventricular canal. J Pediatr 1999;135:703–6.

[11] Jhang WK, Choi J-H, Lee BH, Kim G-H, Yoo H-W. Cardiac manifestations and associations with gene mutations in patients diagnosed with RASopathies. Pediatr Cardiol 2016;37:1539–47.

[12] Colquitt JL, Noonan JA. Cardiac findings in Noonan syndrome on long-term follow-up. Congenit Heart Dis 2014;9:144–50.

[13] Prendiville TW, Gauvreau K, Tworog-Dube E, et al. Cardiovascular disease in Noonan syndrome. Arch Dis Child 2014;99:629–34.

[14] Sznajer Y, Keren B, Baumann C, et al. The spectrum of cardiac anomalies in Noonan syndrome as a result of mutations in the PTPN11 gene. Pediatrics 2007;119(6).

[15] Jongmans M, Sistermans EA, Rikken A, Nillesen WM, Tamminga R, Patton M, Maier EM, Tartaglia M, Noordam K, van der Burgt I. Genotypic and phenotypic characterization of Noonan syndrome: new data and review of the literature. Am J Med Genet A 2005;134:165–70.

[16] Zenker M, Buheitel G, Rauch R, Koenig F, Bosse K, Kress W, Tietze H-U, Doerr H-G, Hofbeck M, Singer H, Reis A, Rauch A. Genotype-phenotype correlations in Noonan syndrome. J Pediatr 2004;144:368–74.

[17] Sarkozy A, Conti E, Seripa D, Digilio MC, Grifone N, Tandoi C, Fazio VM, Di Ciommo V, Marino B, Pizzuti A, Dallapiccola B. Correlation between PTPN11gene mutations and congenital heart defects in Noonan and LEOPARD syndromes. J Med Genet 2003;40:704–8.

[18] Tartaglia M, Kalidas K, Shaw A, Song X, Musat DL, van der Burgt I, Brunner HG, Bertola DR, Crosby A, Ion A, Kucherlapati RS, Jeffery S, Patton MA, Gelb BD. PTPN11 mutations in Noonan syndrome: molecular spectrum, genotype-phenotype correlation, and phenotypic heterogeneity. Am J Hum Genet 2002;70:1555–63.

[19] Noonan JA. Noonan syndrome and related disorders. Prog Pediatr Cardiol 2005;20:177–85.

[20] Shaw AC, Kalidas K, Crosby AH, Jeffery S, Patton MA. The natural history of Noonan syndrome: a long-term follow-up study. Arch Dis Child 2007;92:128–32.

[21] Raaijmakers R, Noordam C, Noonan JA, Croonen EA, van der Burgt CJ, et al. Are ECG abnormalities in Noonan syndrome characteristic for the syndrome? Eur J Pediatr 2008;167:1363–7.

[22] Chen B, Bronson RT, Klaman LD, et al. Mice mutant for Egfr and Shp2 have defective cardiac semilunar valvulogenesis. Nat Genet 2000;24(3):296–9.

[23] Maheshwari M, Belmont J, Fernbach S, et al. PTPN11 mutations in Noonan syndrome type I: detection of recurrent mutations in exons 3 and 13. Hum Mutat 2002;20:298–304.

[24] Aoki Y, Niihori T, Banjo T, Okamoto N, Mizuno S, Kurosawa K, Ogata T, Takada F, Yano M, Ando T, Hoshika T, Barnett C, Ohashi H, Kawame H, Hasegawa T, Okutani T, Nagashima T, Hasegawa S, Funayama R, Nagashima T, Nakayama K, Inoue S, Watanabe Y, Ogura T, Matsubara Y. Gain-of-function mutations in RIT1 cause Noonan syndrome, a RAS/MAPK pathway syndrome. Am J Hum Genet 2013;93:173–80.

[25] Yaoita M, Niihori T, Mizuno S, Okamoto N, Hayashi S, Watanabe A, Yokozawa M, Suzumura H, Nakahara A, Nakano Y, Hokosaki T, Ohmori A, Sawada H, Migita O, Mima A, Lapunzina P, Santos-Simarro F, GarcíaMiñaúr S, Ogata T, Kawame H, Kurosawa K, Ohashi H, Inoue S, Matsubara Y, Kure S, Aoki Y. Spectrum of mutations and genotype-phenotype analysis in Noonan syndrome patients with RIT1 mutations. Hum Genet 2016;135:209–22.

[26] Roberts AE, Araki T, Swanson KD, Montgomery KT, Schiripo TA, Joshi VA, Li L, Yassin Y, Tamburino AM, Neel BG, Kucherlapati RS. Germline gain-of-function mutations in SOS1 cause Noonan syndrome. Nat Genet 2007;39:70–4.

[27] Lo FS, Lin JL, Kuo MT, et al. Noonan syndrome caused by germline KRAS mutation in Taiwan: report of two patients and a review of the literature. Eur J Pediatr 2009;168:919–23.

[28] Cordeddu V, Di Schiavi E, Pennacchio LA, Ma'ayan A, Sarkozy A, et al. Mutation of SHOC2 promotes aberrant protein N-myristoylation and causes Noonan-like syndrome with loose anagen hair. Nat Genet 2009;41:1022–6.

[29] Iacobazzi D, Garaeva I, Albertario A, Cherif M, Angelini GD, Caputo M, Ghorbel MT. Protein phosphatase 1 beta is modulated by chronic hypoxia and involved in the angiogenic endothelial cell migration. Cell Physiol Biochem 2015;36:384–94.

[30] Liu R, Correll RN, Davis J, Vagnozzi RJ, York AJ, Sargent MA, Naim AC, Molkentin JD. Cardiac-specific deletion of protein phosphatase 1beta promotes increased myofilament protein phosphorylation and contractile alterations. J Mol Cell Cardiol 2015;87:204–13.

[31] Rao PS. Percutaneous balloon pulmonary valvuloplasty: state of the art. Catheter Cardiovasc Interv 2007;69:747–63.

[32] Rao PS, Galal O, Patnana M, et al. Results of three to 10 year follow up of balloon dilatation of the pulmonary valve. Heart 1998;80:591–5.

[33] Hickey EJ, Mehta R, Elmi M, Asoh K, McCrindle BW, Williams WG, Manlhiot C, Benson L. Survival implications: hypertrophic cardiomyopathy in Noonan syndrome. Congenit Heart Dis 2011;6:41–7.

[34] Wilkinson JD, Lowe AM, Salbert BA, et al. Outcomes in children with Noonan syndrome and hypertrophic cardiomyopathy: a study from the Pediatric Cardiomyopathy Registry. Am Heart J 2012;164:442–8.

[35] Sharland M, Burch M, McKenna WM, Patton MA. A clinical study of Noonan syndrome. Arch Dis Child 1992;67(2):178–83.

[36] Saccà L, Napoli R, Cittadini A. Growth hormone, acromegaly, and heart failure: an intricate triangulation. Clin Endocrinol 2003;59:660–71.

[37] Cotterill AM, McKenna WJ, Brady AF, et al. The short-term effects of growth hormone therapy on height velocity and cardiac ventricular wall thickness in children with Noonan's syndrome. J Clin Endocrinol Metab 1996;81:2291–7.

[38] Romano AA, Blethen SL, Dana K, Noto RA. Growth hormone treatment in Noonan syndrome: the National Cooperative Growth Study experience. J Pediatr 1996;128: S18–21.

[39] Romano AA, Dana K, Bakker B, et al. Growth response, near-adult height, and patterns of growth and puberty in patients with Noonan syndrome treated with growth hormone. J Clin Endocrinol Metab 2009;94:2338–44.

[40] Noordam C, Draaisma JM, van den Nieuwenhof J. Effects of growth hormone treatment on left ventricular dimensions in children with Noonan's syndrome. Horm Res 2001;56:110–3.

[41] Noordam C, Peer PG, Francois I, De Schepper J, van den Burgt I, Otten BJ. Long-term GH treatment improves adult height in children with Noonan syndrome with and without mutations in protein tyrosine phosphatase, non-receptor-type 11. Eur J Endocrinol 2008;159:203–8.

[42] Otten B, Noordam C. Short stature in Noonan syndrome: Results of growth hormone treatment in KIGS. In: Ranke M, Price D, Reiter E, editors. Growth hormone therapy in pediatrics – 20 years of KIGS. Basel: Karger; 2007. p. 347–55.

[43] Zavras N, Meazza C, Pilotta A, et al. Five-year response to growth hormone in children with Noonan syndrome and growth hormone deficiency. Ital J Pediatr 2015;41:71.

CHAPTER 4

Endocrinopathies Associated With Noonan Syndrome

Sunil K. Sinha*, Alicia Diaz-Thomas[†,‡]

*Department of Endocrinology and Diabetes, Nationwide Children's Hospital, Columbus, OH, United States
[†]Department of Pediatrics, University of Tennessee Health Science Center, Memphis, TN, United States
[‡]LeBonheur Children's Hospital, Memphis, TN, United States

Abstract

Noonan syndrome (NS) is a relatively common autosomal dominant, heterogeneous disorder included in the RASopathies. NS can present with an array of endocrine manifestations. Short stature is one of the cardinal features of NS, which is widely studied and treated. The precise mechanism of other endocrine disorders, such as cryptorchidism, delayed puberty, male infertility are not well delineated. In recent years, our understating of RASopathies' consequences at the cellular level has broadened research and interest in many of these poorly understood manifestations. Effects of the Ras-mitogen-activated protein kinase (MAPK) signaling pathway on bone health, insulin resistance, and metabolism are new areas of interest. This chapter aims to provide a comprehensive review of endocrine manifestation of NS based on current published literatures.

Keywords: Noonan, RASopathies, *PTPN11* gene, MAPK signaling, Short stature, Cryptorchidism, Endocrinopathies, Infertility

Abbreviations

GH	growth hormone
IGF-1	insulin like growth factor-1
***PTPN11* gene**	protein tyrosine phosphatase, nonreceptor type 11
rhGH	recombinant human growth hormone
SHP2	Src-homology 2 domain-containing phosphatase 2 (SHP2)

INTRODUCTION

Noonan syndrome (NS, MIM 163950), a clinically and genetically heterogeneous syndrome, belongs to the RASopathies. These conditions involve activating mutations in genes of the Ras–mitogen–activated protein kinase (MAPK) signaling pathway, an essential pathway for regulation of the cell cycle as well as cell differentiation, growth, migration, and adhesion [1]. NS is a relatively common autosomal dominant disorder with an incidence ranging from 1/1000 to 1/2500 depending upon studies and population evaluated [2]. It is characterized by distinctive facial features (ptosis, hypertelorism, down-slanting palpebral fissures, posteriorly rotated low-set ears), short stature, pubertal delay, cryptorchidism, congenital heart diseases, and an increased risk of certain malignancies [2, 3]. In 2001, Tartaglia et al. first described a mutation in *PTPN11* gene on chromosome 12 as the NS causing molecular alteration, which now comprises about 50% of genetically confirmed cases [4]. The *PTPN11* gene encodes the nonreceptor protein tyrosine phosphatase SHP-2 which positively modulates RAS function. Several other genes have been associated with Noonan syndrome including *KRAS, SOS1, RAF1, BRAF, SHOC2, NRAS, MEK1, RIT1*, and *CBL*. To date, molecular testing can diagnose up to 70% of the Noonan syndrome leaving another 30% having an unidentified genetic makeup which remains to be elucidated.

The phenotype of NS is diverse, and the heterogeneity of clinical presentation is not only limited to the corresponding genotype but also can vary with identical genetic alterations in families. Facial features evolve with age from the newborn period to adulthood making it even harder to identify undiagnosed cases [5]. A number of other overlapping syndromes such as Costello syndrome (CS, MIM # 218040), LEOPARD syndrome (LS, MIM # 151100) and cardio-facio-cutaneous syndrome (CFCS, MIM # 115150) share facial features that need to be considered when evaluating for NS [2].

Endocrine aspects of NS are primarily focused on short stature as it is often described as one of the cardinal features of this entity. Short stature associated with NS is one of the few FDA approved indications for recombinant human growth hormone (rhGH) use. However, the impact of abnormal MAPK signaling pathway on endocrine system, which includes undescended testis, delayed puberty, infertility, autoimmune thyroiditis, bone health and dysmetabolism remains either mostly poorly studied or poorly characterized although associations are evident in medical literature. This review aims to present the current knowledge of endocrine manifestations of NS based on current literature search (Table 1).

GROWTH AND GROWTH HORMONE

Approximately 50%–70% of individuals with NS have short stature, although patient with SOS1 mutations are less likely to be short from genetic potential compared to mutations in PTPN11 [2, 6]. Final adult height in a

Table 1 Endocrinological abnormalities in Noonan syndrome

	Proposed pathophysiology	Provocative testing	Lab findings	Manifestation	Ref.
Growth	GH insensitivity	IGF generation test	Low IGF-1, ALS. Normal IGFBP-3	Short stature	[8, 9, 11]
Thyroid	Autoimmune thyroid disease		Positive anti-TPO and anti-Tg, elevated TSH, low T4, low T3	Mostly euthyroid, acquired hypothyroidism	[15, 36, 37]
Testicular function	Mixed review No effect		Normal LH level, normal testosterone	Pubertal delay Normal-subnormal	[2] [17, 19, 21, 22]
	Compromised gonadal function	HCG stimulation test	Poor testosterone response	Leydig cell function	[13, 20]
		LH-RH stimulation test	Elevated FSH and exaggerated response	Sertoli cell failure, small testicular size during puberty	[13, 17, 21–23]
	Oligospermia, azoospermia		Low AMH and inhibin B Elevated FSH Low inhibin B	Fertility compromised	[17, 19, 20, 23, 31, 32]
Ovaries	Limited information			Pubertal delay	[2]
Bone metabolism	Ras–MAPK antagonize osteogenic differentiation Increased bone turnover		Collagen breakdown product Deoxypyridinoline/ Pyridinoline ratios elevated	Decreased bone mineral density	[38]
Pituitary	Normal			None	[33]
Glucose metabolism	Insulin resistance			~17% impaired glucose tolerance	[34, 35]
Endocrine neoplasm	Higher neoplastic risk			No routine surveillance recommended Cautious rhGH therapy use	[44, 45]

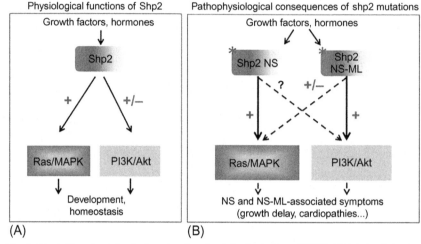

Fig. 1 Model for physiological and pathophysiological roles of SHP2. (A) In physiological conditions, SHP2 participates in the activation of the RAS/MAPK cascade, while it can inhibit or activate the PI3K/AKT pathway. This combined regulation is necessary for proper development and homeostasis. (B) NS-causing SHP2's mutants hyperactivate the RAS/MAPK pathway while the NS-ML-associated mutants hyperactivate the PI3K/AKT pathway. These signaling imbalances are linked to the development of some symptoms of the diseases (cardiopathies, cranio-facial defects, growth delay). NS-ML-linked mutants can also positively or negatively impact the RAS/MAPK pathway, through mechanisms that are poorly understood. *Reproduced from Tajan M, de Rocca Serra A, Valet P, Edouard T, Yart A. SHP2 sails from physiology to pathology. Eur J Med Genet 2015;58(10):509-25. doi: 10.1016/j.ejmg.2015.08.005 with permission from Elsevier.*

NS individual with a PTPN11 mutation is approximately 4 cm less than those without a mutation in both sexes, but the difference was not statistically significant in a study of UK population [7]. Postnatal growth failure is multifactorial in NS and one of mechanisms of *PTPN11* gene mutations, resulting in altered activity of tyrosine phosphatase SHP2 protein. In most cases the overall result is inhibition of insulin-like growth factor 1 (IGF-1) release via growth hormone (GH) induced Ras/mitogen-activated protein kinase (ERK1/2) pathway hyperactivation, and some degree of GH insensitivity [8, 9] (see Fig. 1). Similar mechanism has been proposed to explain the signaling of various other hormones as well. Most children with NS demonstrated varying degree of GH resistance. IGF-1 generation test in a small cohort with PTPN11 mutation showed significantly lower IGF-1 level post generation test (0.05 mg/kg/day for 4 days) when compared to age matched prepubertal short statured children supported presence of some degree of GH resistance [10]. Like IGF-1, acid-labile subunit (ALS) also noted to be very low but IGF-binding protein-3 (IGFBP-3) level is in the normal range for the age and gender [11]. The rhGH use in NS has been approved by the Food and Drug Administration in 2007, however has not been approved by the European Medicines Agency. Response to rhGH therapy is noticeably similar (+1.4 SDS at near-adult height) to that seen in Turner syndrome (+1.2 SDS at near-adult height) although significantly less than isolated growth hormone deficiency (+1.7 SDS at near-adult height) as reported in the National Cooperative Growth Study (NCGS) postmarketing observational study [12].

HYPOTHALAMIC/PITUITARY/GONADAL AXIS

Very limited systematic evaluation of the hypothalamic/pituitary/gonadal axis in patients with NS exists in literature. Available information points to a variable phenotype including but not limited to cryptorchidism, primary gonadal failure, delayed puberty, oligospermia, and azoospermia leading to male infertility. Interestingly, with the exception of delayed puberty, females with NS seem to be spared from gonadal disruptions [2].

Pubertal Development

Although precise etiology is not well elucidated, pubertal delay in NS has been reported in both genders when compared to the general population. Mean age of children with NS entering puberty is between 13.5 and 14.5 years for males and 13 and 14 years for females [2]. The majority achieves delayed but spontaneous puberty; only about 6% of the adolescents with NS required induction of puberty in one study [7]. Theintz et al. described three out of five evaluated patients requiring induction of puberty [13]. Rapid progression of pubertal tempo following delayed initiation is an interesting observation [12]. It is worth noting that, like the general population, delayed puberty can negatively impact bone mass and add a psychosocial burden in individual with syndrome associated multiple stigmata [14].

GONAD AND GONADAL FUNCTION

The prevalence of cryptorchidism is as high as 77% in NS, although location of the gonads are not uniformly described and may affect one or both testes [15]. In general, the etiology of cryptorchidism is thought to be multifactorial: it can be due to a disruption of critical steps during anatomical descent in fetal life, a suboptimal hormonal influence during critical period in gestation, environmental disruption, and/or genetic alteration. Insulin–like hormone 3 (INSL3) and testosterone play pivotal roles in testicular descent directly and indirectly via a neurotransmitter like calcitonin gene-related peptide (CGRP) from hormonal aspect [16]. Currently no systematic study has elucidated the etiology of the high incidence of cryptorchidism in this population. Recently primary gonadal dysfunction has been postulated as a leading cause [13, 17, 18].

The degree of virilization of external genitalia is not well characterized in literature beside undescended testicles (cryptorchidism). Penile length appears to be shorter than average and micopenis had been observed [19].

The assessment of gonadal function in NS is confounded by limited systematic studies but also often by the contradictory findings, likely reflecting the phenotypic heterogeneity in this population. Recent studies on SHP2 knock out transgenic mice demonstrated PTPN11 plays an important role in steroidogenesis, proliferation of spermatogonial stem cells [18]. Okuyama et al. and Theintz et al. both described two subjects each with adequate response to a formal human chorionic gonadotropin (HCG) stimulation test, however five patients and one patient in each respective study showed minimal response [13, 20]. Two separate studies involving three patients aged ranging from 10 to 17 years, demonstrated a normal response to HCG stimulation test [21, 22]. Normal or subnormal Leydig cell function has been reported in several studies based on normal testosterone and LH level [17, 19]. Most studies invariably showed elevated FSH level and an execrated response to luteinizing hormone-releasing hormone (LH-RH) stimulation test also is noted in few studies [13, 17, 22]. Testosterone level is noted in the normal range during pubertal development despite these reported disturbances of the LH function in some function.

Although some disagreements regarding early Leydig cell function exists in scientific literature, poor Sertoli cell function is now rather well documented by the evidence of suppressed antimullerian hormone (AMH) and inhibin B levels: both of which are well established surrogate markers of Sertoli cell function by several studies [17, 21–23].

Testicular volume appears to be small during puberty; however, normalized by adulthood [23]. This smaller volume may be perhaps due to Sertoli cell dysfunction, as Sertoli cells comprise the bulk of the expanding seminiferous tubules responsible for testicular volume at prepubertal age [24, 25].

FERTILITY

Though it has been frequently stated that the cryptorchidism is the cause of infertility in males with NS, more recent studies shed some light on this aspect and broaden the horizon to primary gonadal failure, specifically Sertoli cell dysfunction. Previous studies suggested cryptorchidism itself and timing of the orchidopexy both influence the fertility [26]. Most recent guidelines for management of cryptorchidism from the American Urological Association published in 2014 recommend orchidopexy before 18 months of age to preserve their capacity of steroidogenesis and spermatogenesis and facilitate cancer surveillance [27]. Most cases with NS reporting the timing of the orchidopexy are noted to be beyond the age of current recommendation [17]. However, that NS patients with and without cryptorchidism both have impaired fertility signifies primary gonadal failure as a contributing factor [13]. Sertoli cell dysfunction now appears to be a new point of interest, nonetheless the implication of cryptorchidism itself should be taken into consideration. Mature Sertoli cells create the blood-testis barrier (BTB) to provide adequate microenvironments for spermatogenesis and to secrete several key functional products such as glial cell line-derived neurotrophic factor (GDNF), stem cell factor (SCF), fibroblast growth factor 2 (FGF2), important in germ cell development [28]. Inhibin B, a product of Sertoli cell, has been considered as a marker of impaired fertility and oligospermia; the gradual decline of inhibin B level with pubertal progression leading to impaired negative feedback on FSH and ultimately elevated above age specific normal level [17, 23]. In transgenic mouse model, it has been shown that loss of SHP2 may lead to dysfunctional BTB, an arrest of proliferation of spermatogonial stem cells (SSCs) and decreased renewal for replenishment of SSCs leading to Sertoli cell only type male infertility [29, 30]. Clinically, oligospermia and azoospermia are often accompanied by an immature appearance of Sertoli cells, reduced diameter of seminiferous tubules, interstitial fibrosis and hypospermatogenesis on testicular biopsy [19, 20, 31, 32].

HYPOPITUITARISM/HYPOTHALAMIC AXIS

Although panhypopituitarism reported in a 37 year-old patient, evidence supporting primary pituitary dysfunction associated with NS is lacking [33].

INSULIN RESISTANCE/METABOLIC SYNDROME

Less information is available regarding the metabolic aspects of NS. Lower BMI is a relatively common finding in NS and other RASopathies, and a relative leanness is maintained through adulthood. In one study, impaired glucose tolerance was diagnosed in 17% of patients with NS despite normal range BMI SDS, normal fasting glucose and normal insulin levels. As RAS/MAPK-related proteins seem to have a role in insulin signaling through PI3K/AKT pathway, patients with NS should be considered at risk for developing insulin resistance and its associated complications [34, 35].

AUTOIMMUNE THYROID DISEASE (ATD)

A prospective study done by Quaio et al. showed two-to-three fold increased risk of autoimmune disorders in NS when compared to the general population [36]. Incidence of antithyroid antibodies (antimicrosomal or anti-TPO, antithyroglobulin antibody) are higher among the NS population and range between 30% and 60%, depending on studies. A caveat exists that contradictory results are reported in literature regarding incidence of autoimmune hypothyroidism [15, 36, 37].

As per the Noonan syndrome clinical management guidelines, it is recommended to screen blood for thyroid abnormalities every 3–5 years in older children and adults. Manage abnormalities as in general population with thyroid replacement therapy [2].

Various auto-antibodies were tested and were found to be positive in about 50% of the patients with NS. These antibodies included Antinuclear antibodies, antidouble stranded DNA, anti-SS-A/Ro, anti-SS-B/La, anti-Sm, anti-RNP, anti-Scl-70, anti-Jo-1, antiribosomal P, IgG and IgM anticardiolipin (aCL), thyroid, antismooth muscle, antiendomysial (AE), antiliver cytosolic protein type 1 (LC1), antiparietal cell (APC), antimitochondrial (AM) antibodies, antiliver-kidney microsome type 1 antibodies (LKM-1), and lupus anticoagulant. Only 14% of the patients had fulfilled the criteria for autoimmune disease while about half had some antibodies positive [36].

BONE METABOLISM

Very sparse literature is available on bone health in NS although increased bone turnover and decreased bone mineral density in other RASopathy disorders like neurofibromatosis type 1 (NF1) and Costello syndrome are common. The phenotypic presentation of short stature and skeletal deformities (e.g., pectus, scoliosis) in NS also indicates presence of underlying pathology. In a small cohort, Choudhry et al. showed that children with NS also have a significantly lower total body bone mineral density (BMD) compared to their age, gender, ethnicity, and height matched controls without any significant change of biological markers of bone metabolism [38]. A recent study of patients with NS purported that rather than decrease bone mass caused by secondary risk factors associated with NS, primary bone quality impairment was the culprit in lower bone mass [39]. Deoxypyridinoline (Dpd), a collagen breakdown product, and the deoxypyridinoline/pyridinoline (Dpd/Pyd) ratios were significantly elevated in a small cohort of 14 patients with NS compared to the controls indicating increased bone turnover [40]. Age of onset of puberty itself is an independent predictor of bone mass in young adults and in general may also be a contributing factor [14]. Controversy surrounds Ras signaling in osteogenic processes: Ras-MAPK signals may be essential for the commitment of multipotent progenitors to an osteoblast cell fate, yet they may antagonize further osteogenic differentiation [41]. Thus, it seems that the etiology of the bony phenotype resulting from these processes will require further investigation to unravel.

ENDOCRINE NEOPLASM

NS has been linked with higher risk for benign and malignant proliferative disorders with an incidence rate varying from 3.5 to 8.1-folds depending on various studies; however, tumor surveillance is not recommended by the authors from a recent study evaluating cancer risk in this population [42, 43]. Endocrine neoplasms are rare and are limited to germ cell tumor and adrenal neuroblastoma. There are several case reports of solid brain tumors in literature which warrant taking appropriate caution and implementing monitoring prior to and during rhGH therapy [44, 45]. To date Sertoli cell tumors are reported only in two cases; one case involves 7-year-old clinically diagnosed NS with history of cryptorchidism and the other with proven SOS1 mutation [46, 47].

CONCLUSION

Beside management of short stature associated with NS, pediatricians should therefore be aware of the risk for several endocrinopathies and their manifestations. Understanding the underlying mechanism and natural history of these disorders will help clinicians to formulate appropriate management plan and provide proper counseling of this heterogeneous disease.

REFERENCES

[1] Noonan JA, Ehmke DA. Associated noncardiac malformations in children with congenital heart disease. J Pediatr 1963;63:468–70.

[2] Romano AA, Allanson JE, Dahlgren J, Gelb BD, Hall B, Pierpont ME, et al. Noonan syndrome: clinical features, diagnosis, and management guidelines. Pediatrics 2010;126 (4):746–59.

[3] Mendez HM, Opitz JM. Noonan syndrome: a review. Am J Med Genet 1985;21 (3):493–506.

[4] Tartaglia M, Kalidas K, Shaw A, Song X, Musat DL, van der Burgt I, et al. PTPN11 mutations in Noonan syndrome: molecular spectrum, genotype-phenotype correlation, and phenotypic heterogeneity. Am J Hum Genet 2002;70(6):1555–63.

[5] Allanson JE, Hall JG, Hughes HE, Preus M, Witt RD. Noonan syndrome: the changing phenotype. Am J Med Genet 1985;21(3):507–14.

[6] Tartaglia M, Pennacchio LA, Zhao C, Yadav KK, Fodale V, Sarkozy A, et al. Gain-of-function SOS1 mutations cause a distinctive form of Noonan syndrome. Nat Genet 2007;39(1):75–9.

[7] Shaw AC, Kalidas K, Crosby AH, Jeffery S, Patton MA. The natural history of Noonan syndrome: a long-term follow-up study. Arch Dis Child 2007;92(2):128–32.

[8] Binder G, Neuer K, Ranke MB, Wittekindt NE. PTPN11 mutations are associated with mild growth hormone resistance in individuals with Noonan syndrome. J Clin Endocrinol Metab 2005;90(9):5377–81.

[9] De Rocca S-NA, Edouard T, Treguer K, Tajan M, Araki T, Dance M, et al. Noonan syndrome-causing SHP2 mutants inhibit insulin-like growth factor 1 release via growth hormone-induced ERK hyperactivation, which contributes to short stature. Proc Natl Acad Sci U S A 2012;109(11):4257–62.

[10] Bertelloni S, Baroncelli GI, Dati E, Ghione S, Baldinotti F, Toschi B, et al. IGF-I generation test in prepubertal children with Noonan syndrome due to mutations in the PTPN11 gene. Hormones (Athens) 2013;12(1):86–92.

[11] Limal JM, Parfait B, Cabrol S, Bonnet D, Leheup B, Lyonnet S, et al. Noonan syndrome: relationships between genotype, growth, and growth factors. J Clin Endocrinol Metab 2006;91(1):300–6.

[12] Romano AA, Dana K, Bakker B, Davis DA, Hunold JJ, Jacobs J, et al. Growth response, near-adult height, and patterns of growth and puberty in patients with Noonan syndrome treated with growth hormone. J Clin Endocrinol Metab 2009;94(7):2338–44.

[13] Theintz G, Savage MO. Growth and pubertal development in five boys with Noonan's syndrome. Arch Dis Child 1982;57(1):13–7.

[14] Gilsanz V, Chalfant J, Kalkwarf H, Zemel B, Lappe J, Oberfield S, et al. Age at onset of puberty predicts bone mass in young adulthood. J Pediatr 2011;158(1):100–5, 105. e1–2.

[15] Sharland M, Burch M, McKenna WM, Paton MA. A clinical study of Noonan syndrome. Arch Dis Child 1992;67(2):178–83.

[16] Hutson JM, Southwell BR, Li R, Lie G, Ismail K, Harisis G, et al. The regulation of testicular descent and the effects of cryptorchidism. Endocr Rev 2013;34(5):725–52.

[17] Marcus KA, Sweep CG, van der Burgt I, Noordam C. Impaired Sertoli cell function in males diagnosed with Noonan syndrome. J Pediatr Endocrinol Metab 2008;21 (11):1079–84.

[18] Puri P, Walker WH. The regulation of male fertility by the PTPN11 tyrosine phosphatase. Semin Cell Dev Biol 2016;59:27–34. https://doi.org/10.1016/j. semcdb.2016.01.020.

[19] Elsawi MM, Pryor JP, Klufio G, Barnes C, Patton MA. Genital tract function in men with Noonan syndrome. J Med Genet 1994;31(6):468–70.

[20] Okuyama A, Nishimoto N, Yoshioka T, Namiki M, Itatani H, Takaha M, et al. Gonadal findings in cryptorchid boys with Noonan's phenotype. Eur Urol 1981;7 (5):274–7.

[21] Saez JM, Morera AM, Bertrand J. Testicular endocrine function in males with Noonan's syndrome. Lancet 1969;2(7629):1078–9.

[22] Kauschansky A, Eilam N, Elian E. LH-RH and HCG studies in a turner phenotype male (Noonan's syndrome). A case report. Helv Paediatr Acta 1977;32(3):237–40.

[23] Ankarberg-Lindgren C, Westphal O, Dahlgren J. Testicular size development and reproductive hormones in boys and adult males with Noonan syndrome: a longitudinal study. Eur J Endocrinol 2011;165(1):137–44.

[24] Nistal M, Abaurrea MA, Paniagua R. Morphological and histometric study on the human Sertoli cell from birth to the onset of puberty. J Anat 1982;134(Pt 2):351–63.

[25] Cortes D, Muller J, Skakkebaek NE. Proliferation of Sertoli cells during development of the human testis assessed by stereological methods. Int J Androl 1987;10(4):589–96.

[26] Hadziselimovic F, Hocht B, Herzog B, Buser MW. Infertility in cryptorchidism is linked to the stage of germ cell development at orchidopexy. Horm Res 2007;68 (1):46–52.

[27] Kolon TF, Herndon CD, Baker LA, Baskin LS, Baxter CG, Cheng EY, et al. Evaluation and treatment of cryptorchidism: AUA guideline. J Urol 2014;192(2):337–45.

[28] Mital P, Hinton BT, Dufour JM. The blood-testis and blood-epididymis barriers are more than just their tight junctions. Biol Reprod 2011;84(5):851–8.

[29] Puri P, Phillips BT, Suzuki H, Orwig KE, Rajkovic A, Lapinski PE, et al. The transition from stem cell to progenitor spermatogonia and male fertility requires the SHP2 protein tyrosine phosphatase. Stem Cells 2014;32(3):741–53.

[30] Hu X, Tang Z, Li Y, Liu W, Zhang S, Wang B, et al. Deletion of the tyrosine phosphatase Shp2 in Sertoli cells causes infertility in mice. Sci Rep 2015;5:12982.

[31] Nistal M, Paniagua R, Pallardo LF. Testicular biopsy and hormonal study in a male with Noonan's syndrome. Andrologia 1983;15(5):415–25.

[32] Sasagawa I, Nakada T, Kubota Y, Sawamura T, Tateno T, Ishigooka M. Gonadal function and testicular histology in Noonan's syndrome with bilateral cryptorchidism. Arch Androl 1994;32(2):135–40.

[33] Ross JL, Shenkman L. Noonan's syndrome and hypopituitarism. Am J Med Sci 1980;279(1):47–52.

[34] Boucher J, Kleinridders A, Kahn CR. Insulin receptor signaling in normal and insulin-resistant states. Cold Spring Harb Perspect Biol 2014;6(1):1–23.

[35] Malaquias AC, Couto XC, Moraes MB, Funari MF, Pereira AC, Villares SM, et al. In: Metabolic profile in patients with Noonan and Noonan-like syndromes suggests a role of RAS/MAPK pathway mutations in insulin signaling. Endocrine Society's 97th Annual Meeting and Expo; March 5; San Diego, CA; 2015.

[36] Quaio CR, Carvalho JF, da Silva CA, Bueno C, Brasil AS, Pereira AC, et al. Autoimmune disease and multiple autoantibodies in 42 patients with RASopathies. Am J Med Genet A 2012;158A(5):1077–82.

[37] Vesterhus P, Aarskog D. Noonan's syndrome and autoimmune thyroiditis. J Pediatr 1973;83(2):237–40.

[38] Choudhry KS, Grover M, Tran AA, O'Brian Smith E, Ellis KJ, Lee BH. Decreased bone mineralization in children with Noonan syndrome: another consequence of dysregulated RAS MAPKinase pathway? Mol Genet Metab 2012;106(2):237–40.

[39] Baldassarre G, Mussa A, Carli D, Molinatto C, Ferrero GB. Constitutional bone impairment in Noonan syndrome. Am J Med Genet A 2017;173(3):692–8.

[40] Stevenson DA, Schwarz EL, Carey JC, Viskochil DH, Hanson H, Bauer S, et al. Bone resorption in syndromes of the Ras/MAPK pathway. Clin Genet 2011;80(6):566–73.

[41] Schindeler A, Little DG. Ras MAPK signaling in osteogenic differentiation: friend or foe? J Bone Miner Res 2006;21(9):1331–8.

[42] Kratz CP, Franke L, Peters H, Kohlschmidt N, Kazmierczak B, Finckh U, et al. Cancer spectrum and frequency among children with Noonan, Costello, and cardio-facio-cutaneous syndromes. Br J Cancer 2015;112(8):1392–7.

[43] Jongmans MC, van der Burgt I, Hoogerbrugge PM, Noordam K, Yntema HG, Nillesen WM, et al. Cancer risk in patients with Noonan syndrome carrying a PTPN11 mutation. Eur J Hum Genet 2011;19(8):870–4.

[44] Bangalore Krishna K, Pagan P, Escobar O, Popovic J. Occurrence of cranial neoplasms in pediatric patients with Noonan syndrome receiving growth hormone: is screening with brain MRI prior to initiation of growth hormone indicated? Horm Res Paediatr 2017;88(6):423–6.

[45] Siegfried A, Cances C, Denuelle M, Loukh N, Tauber M, Cave H, et al. Noonan syndrome, PTPN11 mutations, and brain tumors. A clinical report and review of the literature. Am J Med Genet A 2017;173(4):1061–5.

[46] Fryssira H, Leventopoulos G, Psoni S, Kitsiou-Tzeli S, Stavrianeas N, Kanavakis E. Tumor development in three patients with Noonan syndrome. Eur J Pediatr 2008;167(9):1025–31.

[47] Denayer E, Devriendt K, de Ravel T, Van Buggenhout G, Smeets E, Francois I, et al. Tumor spectrum in children with Noonan syndrome and SOS1 or RAF1 mutations. Genes Chromosom Cancer 2010;49(3):242–52.

CHAPTER 5

Genitourinary Manifestation of Noonan Syndrome

Peter Zhan Tao Wang*, Francisco J. Garcia†, Elias Wehbi‡
*Western University, London, ON, Canada
†Cypress Regional Hospital, Swift Current, SK, Canada
‡University of California, Irvine, CA, United States

Abstract

Noonan syndrome is a rare and dynamic condition that commonly affects the genitourinary system. This chapter will discuss the common genitourinary manifestations of Noonan syndrome. These manifestations include abnormalities to the kidneys, testicles, scrotum, and with future fertility. In this chapter, the diagnosis, management, and prognosis of each of these manifestations will be detailed.

Keywords: Urology, Noonan, Genitourinary, Management, Pediatric

Abbreviations

AD-S	adult dark-spermatogonia
APD	anteroposterior diameter
AR	androgen receptor
AUA	American Urological Association
CGRP	calcitonin gene–related peptide
CUA	Canadian Urological Association
EUA	European Urological Association
FSH	follicle stimulating hormone
GFN	genitofemoral nerve
GnRH	gonadotropin-releasing hormone
GU	genitourinary
HCG	human chorionic gonadotropin
ICSI	intracytoplasmic sperm injection
INSL3	insulin-like hormone 3
IVF	in-vitro fertilization
LH	luteinizing hormone
LH-RH	luteinizing releasing hormone
MIS	Mullerian-inhibiting substance
NPO	nothing by mouth
NS	Noonan syndrome
SFU	Society of Fetal Urology
UDT	undescended testis
β-HCG	beta human chorionic gonadotropin

Noonan Syndrome
https://doi.org/10.1016/B978-0-12-815348-2.00004-9

INTRODUCTION

Dr. Jacqueline Noonan first described Noonan syndrome (NS) in a case series of nine patients with pulmonary valve stenosis, small stature, hypertelorism, mild intellectual disability, ptosis, undescended testes, and skeletal malformations [1, 2]. The incidence of NS is 1 per 1000–2500 live births without gender predominance [3]. It is autosomal dominant with multiple congenital abnormalities affecting numerous systems, including the genitourinary system. In this chapter, these genitourinary abnormalities, including their diagnosis and management, will be discussed.

PATHOPHYSIOLOGY

This heterogeneous condition is associated with several genetic and molecular abnormalities. NS is associated with mutations in the RAS/MAPK (mitogen-activated protein kinase) signal transduction pathway. Mutations in this pathway are found in 61% of NS patients [3]. This pathway is involved in cellular proliferation, differentiation, and apoptosis. Overall, six relevant genes encoding components of the RAS/MAPK pathway have been identified; most importantly the *PTPN11*, *KRAS*, *SOS1*, *RAF1*, *NRAS*, and *SHOC2* genes [4].

In nearly half of the patients with NS, there is a missense mutation in the *PTPN11* gene. *PTPN11* is located on the long arm of chromosome 12, which codes for the nonreceptor protein tyrosine phosphatase SHP-2 [5, 6]. SHP-2 is involved in different cellular processes during embryonic development. Jongmans et al. identified 19 different missense mutations studying 68 patients with NS. In general, these missense mutations increase SHP-2 activity resulting in increased RAS-MAPK signaling [4, 7].

DIAGNOSIS
Cardinal Characteristics

NS is associated with characteristic facial features such as hypertelorism (65%), downslanting palpebral fissures (96%), ptosis (89%), low set ears (93%), low posterior hairline (68%), and webbing of the neck (29%) [8, 9]. Other cardinal features include short stature (93%), bleeding diathesis, wide-set nipples (43%), pectus excavatum (54%), and congenital heart disease (74%) such as pulmonary valve stenosis [7, 10, 11]. Learning disability is present in 10%–25% of NS patients [9].

In the prenatal period, nonspecific features on ultrasound such as poly-hydramnios, hydronephrosis, hydrothorax, cardiac abnormalities, cystic hygroma, and increased nuchal translucency have been reported [8]. Hydro-thorax is the most common prenatal finding in patients with NS. Further-more, NS has been reported in up to 10% of fetuses with normal chromosomes and cystic hygromas diagnosed in the second trimester.

Genetic Testing

Although NS is an autosomal dominant disorder with complete penetrance, it is clinically heterogonous due to variable expressivity [3]. Traditionally, due to its phenotypic variability, NS was often underdiagnosed. To further complicate things, a characteristic of NS is that the phenotype changes with age [10]. Adult patients with NS have more subtle characteristic facial features.

Genetic testing is widely available and can provide confirmation of NS in 70% of cases [10]. Scenarios where genetic testing is beneficial include patients with mild features, adults with suspected NS and where the specific genotype is required for individualized management [8]. However, despite these advances in our understanding of the genetics behind NS, in 30%–40% of patients with NS, no associated genes have been identified; as such NS remains a clinical diagnosis.

Genitourinary Evaluation and Workup

The initial evaluation requires a thorough history and physical examination. As part of the genitourinary examination, Tanner stage should be described as this is an indication of pubertal development. The genitourinary exam should also include penile stretch length, location of the meatus, circumci-sion status, and presence of penile torque or chordee.

Of particular interest in males with NS is the testicular exam. This should be performed with the child supine and the legs crossed in a frog-legged position. Abducting the thighs inhibits the cremasteric reflex. A bimanual technique is most effective in differentiating a retractile testicle versus a truly undescended testicle. The technique is performed with the nondominant hand gently sweeping down along the inguinal canal while the other hand palpates the scrotum and groin for the testis. The use of lubrication is recom-mended. The examination should document testicular location, mobility, size, nodules, and associated abnormalities such as scrotal symmetry, inguinal hernias, and hydroceles.

Imaging Studies

In obese patients, where the physical exam is equivocal and neither testicle is confidently identified, a scrotal and inguinal ultrasound may be warranted to rule out cryptorchidism. In addition, children with NS should have a renal bladder ultrasound at diagnosis to rule out any renal or bladder abnormalities.

GENITOURINARY ABNORMALITIES

Renal and Bladder Abnormalities

Renal anomalies associated with NS includes solitary kidneys, hydrone-phrosis, and duplicated renal collecting systems. These occur in 10%–11% of children with NS [12], and in one cohort reached 50%. In the prenatal period, 19% of NS pregnancies were associated with pelviectasis, hydrone-phrosis, and renal enlargement [13]. Bladder abnormalities associated with NS are rare. There are few case reports of patients with NS diagnosed with congenital urachal cysts [5].

A study by George et al. reported a frequency of 11% for renal anomalies in patients with NS ($n = 44$), aged 9 months to 38 years old, undergoing sur-veillance abdominal ultrasounds [14]. This is lower than that seen in Turner syndrome. The spectrum of renal anomalies reported ranged from minor abnormalities of rotation to duplex systems, hypoplastic kidneys, bilateral renal cysts, unilateral renal scarring, horseshoe kidneys, and solitary kidneys. The most common anomaly was dilation of the renal pelvis in a pattern resembling a ureteropelvic junction obstruction [14]. In the same study, one of the patients had a combination of an ectopic left kidney, a choledo-chal cyst and a midgut malrotation.

Other rare associations between NS and the genitourinary system include: cake (fused) kidneys [15], crossed fused ectopic kidneys, focal seg-mental glomerulosclerosis leading to nephrotic syndrome [16], bilateral duplicated renal collecting systems [17], bilateral kidney duplications [18], and even cases of renal failure having been reported secondary to renal dysplasia and polycystic disease [19].

In one interesting case report, a 9-year-old girl with NS was identified with an extremely rare urinary anomaly. She had bilateral ectopic upper pole ureteral insertions into the vaginal introitus. She presented with continuous incontinence and was found to have two orifices lateral to the urethra mea-tus. An intravenous pyelogram showed bifid collecting systems bilaterally with double ureters. The patient underwent a pyelopyeloplasty on the left and a heminephrectomy on the right for severe hydronephrosis [20].

Management

Renal bladder ultrasounds should be performed in every child with NS. The management of renal abnormalities depends on the ultrasound findings. In patients with a solitary kidney, referral to both a nephrologist and pediatric urologist should be initiated [3]. These patients require long-term surveillance to ensure good renal function and to prevent renal injury.

Similarly, the management of NS patients with a diagnosis of hydronephrosis or a duplicated renal collecting system should be deferred to a pediatric urologist. It is useful to describe the Society for Fetal Urology (SFU) grade, the anteroposterior diameter (APD), laterality and any associated hydroureter. The appearance of the bladder should also be described. The long-term follow-up of NS patients with these renal abnormalities is scarce. As such, there are currently no syndrome specific treatment guidelines.

The decision to perform a voiding cystogram depends on a number of factors including the degree of hydronephrosis, presence of hydroureter, duplication of the renal collecting system, presentation with a febrile urinary tract infection, gender, and the presence or absence of bladder and bowel dysfunction. If vesicoureteral reflux is found, management should also be deferred to a pediatric urologist. The management of this is complex and beyond the scope of this chapter.

Genital Abnormalities

Cryptorchidism

Cryptorchidism is the most common genital abnormality and is found in 70%–90% of males with NS [3, 5, 21, 22]. Of these, approximately 60% are bilateral [23]. Cryptorchidism or undescended testis (UDT) is defined as the failure of a testis to descend into the base of the scrotum.

Undescended testes are further subclassified into palpable and nonpalpable. An undescended testis that is palpable is in a location distal to the internal inguinal ring. Common locations for palpable undescended testes are shown in Fig. 1. The most common position for a palpable undescended testis is the superficial inguinal pouch, which is medial to the external inguinal ring, and anterior to the rectus abdominus muscle.

Nonpalpable testes are intraabdominal and are located anywhere along the path of normal testicular descent. These are either in the abdomen or in a trans-inguinal "peeping" location. The testis may also be completely

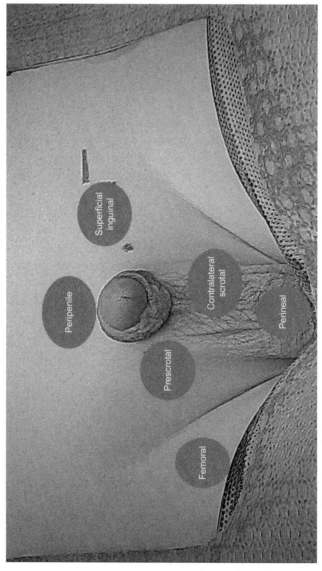

Fig. 1 Most common locations for palpable undescended testes.

atrophic (vanishing testes) or nonpalpable due to an uncooperative patient or due to body habitus. In situations of bilateral nonpalpable undescended testes with abnormal penile development (such as hypospadias), congenital adrenal hyperplasia should be ruled out. Furthermore, chromosomal and hormonal analysis should be performed to rule out a disorder of sexual development.

Pathophysiology

The current knowledge of normal testicular descent is largely extrapolated from animal studies. An intact hypothalamic-pituitary-gonadal axis is essential for normal testicular descent. Prenatal androgen deficiency secondary to insufficient fetal pituitary gonadotropin stimulation or placental gonadotropin is considered the most common cause of cryptorchidism [24]. Fetal gonadotropins such as luteinizing hormone (LH), follicle stimulating hormone (FSH), and beta human chorionic gonadotropin (ß-HCG) regulate the production of androgens, Müllerian-inhibiting substance (MIS) and Insulin-like hormone 3 (INSL3).

Testicular descent is comprised of a transabdominal and inguinoscrotal phase, which are tightly regulated by both anatomical and hormonal factors [21]. In the transabdominal phase, descent of the testis is accomplished by testicular enlargement, mesonephros regression, and the gubernacular swelling reaction. This phase is also regulated by intra-abdominal pressure, as demonstrated by the higher incidence of cryptorchidism in children with abdominal wall defects [21].

Indirect evidence from animal studies have demonstrated that INSL3, secreted by Leydig cells, is a key hormone in the transabdominal phase of testicular descent [25]. The gubernacular swelling reaction, specifically myogenic differentiation of the cremaster, is synergistically controlled by INSL3 and androgens [26]. Furthermore, INSL3 is also involved in the dilatation of the inguinal canal and is required for the expression of androgen receptors (ARs) in the gubernaculum [21].

In the inguinoscrotal phase, the gubernaculum migrates to the scrotum. This phase rarely occurs prior to 22 weeks of gestation and is regulated by androgens via the genitofemoral nerve (GFN) [27]. Studies in animals have demonstrated that calcitonin gene-related peptide (CGRP) released from the GFN is essential for the normal development and function of the gubernaculum [28]. In humans, the cremaster and GFN surround the gubernaculum by 7 weeks gestation [29].

The molecular pathways involved in UDT specific to males with NS remains poorly understood; however, the mechanisms are most likely due to aberrations in several molecular processes involving the RAS/MAPK pathway. SHP-2, the product of the *PTPN11* gene, is known to activate Hoxa-10 [30]. Rijli et al. showed that Hoxa-10 mutant mice exhibited unilateral or bilateral cryptorchidism due to developmental abnormalities of the gubernaculum, further resulting in abnormal spermatogenesis and sterility [31].

Management
In NS males with cryptorchidism, the indications for intervention include improving fertility, decreasing the risk of testicular malignancy, testicular surveillance and cosmesis [21]. Patients with bilateral cryptorchidism have a higher risk of testicular cancer and infertility than those with unilateral disease [32].

The postnatal transformation of neonatal gonocytes into adult dark-spermatogonia (AD-S) is essential for future fertility [21]. AD-S is currently believed to be the putative stem cell necessary for spermatogenesis. This transformation occurs between 3 and 9 months. Normal AD-S development requires strict temperature regulation to ensure it is below that of the body [21]. This is often not possible in an undescended testis. The clinical consequences of this impaired transformation into AD-S leads to poor semen quality and potential risk for infertility.

Elevated environmental temperature has been suggested to be the mechanism by which testicular tumors develop. The relatively higher temperatures prevent gonocyte apoptosis. The persistence of gonocytes coupled with impaired DNA repair leads to a 5–10 × increased risk of testicular cancer [21]. Although intervention decreases this risk and allows for surveillance by physical exam, there is currently no evidence to suggest the risk of testicular cancer is eliminated.

NS patients with cryptorchidism should be referred to a pediatric urologist or an adult urologist depending on the age of the patient for further evaluation and management. Historically, treatment for cryptorchidism was recommended between 1 and 2 years of age based on morphological changes seen on testicular biopsies of undescended testis found on electron microscopy. However, current guidelines recommend intervention between 6–12 months of age [32, 33].

Treatment options include both medical and surgical modalities. However, medical therapy with human chorionic gonadotropin (HCG), gonadotropin-releasing hormone (GnRH), or luteinizing releasing hormone (LH-RH) have a success rate of less than 25% depending on the location of the undescended testis [34]. As such, this is rarely used in current practice and should not be considered a first line treatment for primary UDT.

There is a paucity of studies describing the characteristics of cryptorchidism in NS males. The distribution of NS patients with palpable versus nonpalpable undescended testes is unknown. Furthermore, descriptions regarding the locations of these undescended testes are lacking in the literature.

Surgical intervention for cryptorchidism, as per the American Urological Association (AUA), is recommended by 6–12 months of (corrected gestational) age [32, 33]. Observation is indicated in the first 6 months of life, as the spontaneous rate of testicular descent in patients with cryptorchidism at birth reaches over 50% by 3 months [35]. However, after 6 months, spontaneous testicular descent is unlikely [36]. In addition, a randomized controlled trial by Kollin et al. found improved testicular growth with early surgical intervention at 9 months compared to 3 years of age [37]. Lastly, delaying surgical intervention until after 6 months of age minimizes the risk of general anesthetic to the patient.

Fig. 2 summarizes the general evaluation algorithm for a patient with cryptorchidism. If the testicle is found to be retractile, continued surveillance is advocated to monitor for secondary ascent. The gold standard for the diagnosis of undescended testes requires an examination under anesthesia. If the testis is undescended but palpable, then an inguinal orchidopexy with or without concomitant inguinal hernia repair is the standard of care. A scrotal orchidopexy may be performed in selected cases where the testes are close or can be drawn into the scrotum, and where an inguinal hernia is absent.

If the testis is undescended and nonpalpable on examination under anesthesia, then a diagnostic laparoscopy is indicated. Although an inguinal exploration may be attempted, 23%–38% of patients will require a diagnostic laparoscopy for definitive management [38]. The findings on diagnostic laparoscopy will guide treatment (Fig. 3).

A normal finding includes a closed internal inguinal ring with normal appearing spermatic vessels and vas deferens (Fig. 4). The testis may be intra-abdominal (Fig. 5), inguinal, vanishing or "peeping" in and out of the internal inguinal ring (Fig. 6). If the internal inguinal ring is closed and a normal vas and spermatic vessels are present, then the initial examination may have missed a palpable undescended testis either because it is atrophic, or the patient's body habitus was prohibitory. Atrophic gonadal vessels coursing into a closed internal inguinal ring is suggestive of atrophy (Fig. 7).

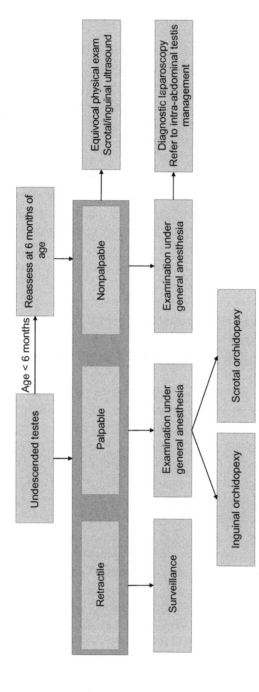

Fig. 2 General evaluation algorithm for a patient with suspected cryptorchidism.

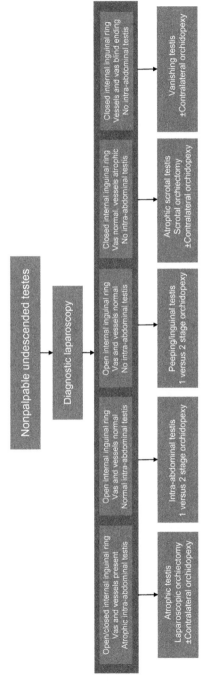

Fig. 3 Treatment algorithm for nonpalpable undescended testes based on diagnostic laparoscopy findings.

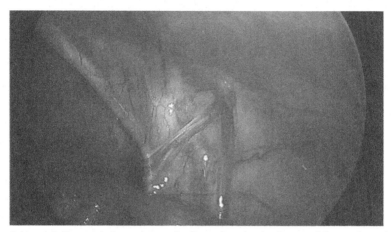

Fig. 4 Normal diagnostic laparoscopy findings showing both gonadal vessels and vas deference entering a closed internal inguinal ring.

Preoperative Care The general health of the patient should be optimized to minimize the risk of general anesthetics, as an orchidopexy is an elective procedure. The patient should be NPO as per institutional guidelines. The patient should also be free from skin infections in the groin area that may affect postoperative healing. Preoperative antibiotics are generally not required unless deemed necessary in the perioperative assessment.

Anatomical Considerations The inguinal anatomy in pediatrics differs from those of adults, especially when operating on infants. The fascia of Camper and Scarpa are thicker and resembles the aponeurosis of the external oblique, which itself is relatively thin [39]. Furthermore, the cremaster is very well developed and blends with the internal oblique. Compared to adults, the course of the inguinal canal in pediatrics is more transverse.

Complications The potential postoperative complications are rare (<1%) and may be categorized into immediate, short-term and long-term. Immediate complications include scrotal swelling, scrotal hematoma, and infection (epididymo-orchitis) [33]. If a scrotal hematoma does not resolve or if it is progressive than surgical intervention may be required. Infections in the immediate period should be treated with antibiotics.

In the short term, patients may develop hydroceles, inadequate testicular position or testicular atrophy. Long-term complications include testicular atrophy or retraction of the testicle. Except for testicular atrophy, which

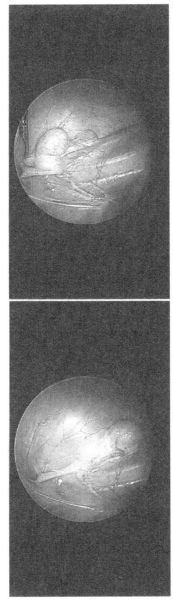

Fig. 5 Diagnostic laparoscopy showing an intra-abdominal testis with an open internal inguinal ring.

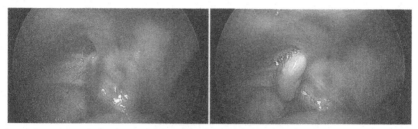

Fig. 6 Diagnostic laparoscopy showing a "peeping" testis.

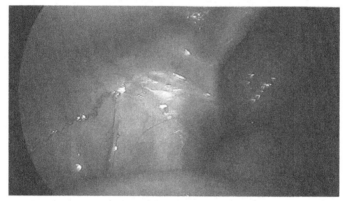

Fig. 7 Diagnostic laparoscopy showing a closed internal inguinal ring with atrophic gonadal vessels suggestive of an atrophic testis in either the inguinal canal or scrotum.

may be due to either inherent or technical factors, a second surgery may be required. Lastly, injury to the vas deferens that is recognized intraoperatively or postoperatively may be repaired immediately or postpuberty with microsurgical techniques.

Orlando et al., reviewing 2650 diagnostic laparoscopies, found a minor complication rate of 1.58% including subcutaneous insufflation [40]. However, other rare, but potential complications of laparoscopy include abdominal wall hematoma, umbilical hernia, bladder injury, bowel injury, and vascular trauma [38].

Other Management Considerations In patients with intra–abdominal testes that are considered too high to treat with a staged procedure, some have advocated a microvascular orchidopexy. However, this technique requires a special skill set and equipment thereby limiting is applicability.

Patients with bilateral UDT pose a special challenge. If both the testes are nonpalpable, MIS levels should be obtained to rule out anorchia [32].

Anecdotally, if the bilateral UDT are palpable then some advocate bilateral procedures during the same general anesthetics. If the bilateral UDT are nonpalpable then each side can be performed at separate times due to the increased risk of testicular atrophy, however this depends on surgeon comfort and experience.

Scrotal Lymphedema

The association between NS and lymphedema is well established. Patients may present with generalized lymphedema, peripheral lymphedema, pulmonary lymphangiectasia, intestinal lymphangiectasia, cystic hygroma, and hydrops fetalis [41]. Approximately 20% of NS patients have peripheral lymphedema [8]. Primary scrotal lymphedema is a rare entity, whereas secondary scrotal lymphedema is a known complication of orchidopexy [42].

It has been postulated that some of the cardinal features of NS may be the direct result of lymphatic obstruction or dysfunction during fetal development [8]. This includes webbing of the neck, hypertelorism, and ptosis. It is even theorized that in-utero lymphedema affects the normal migration of the gonads leading to the anomalous sites of cryptorchidism.

Management

For NS patients suffering from symptomatic scrotal lymphedema, treatment options are limited. Conservative measures such as manual lymphatic drainage and presotherapy have yielded poor results [41]. Surgery involves excision of the affected skin and subcutaneous tissue in a staged manner with or without grafts. The potential complications of these procedures include recurrence of lymphedema, skin necrosis, and severe infections [41]. As such, surgical intervention is reserved for those refractory to conservative management.

Puberty and Fertility

Pubertal patterns vary in NS males and includes normal virilization and fertility, delayed but normal puberty, and inadequate secondary sexual development with deficient spermatogenesis. In males with deficient spermatogenesis, gonadotrophin levels are elevated [11]. The proposed etiologies for this hypergonadotrophic hypogonadism include cryptorchidism, primary gonadal dysfunction with impaired androgen production or panhypopituitarism [7].

Delayed puberty is typically observed in both males and females with NS and characterized by a dampened pubertal growth spurt. The mean age of puberty for boys and girls are 13.5–14.5 and 13–14 years old, respectively [3].

Pathophysiology

Puberty and spermatogenesis are regulated by the male hypothalamo-pituitary-gonadal axis. High levels of Müllerian inhibiting substance (MIS) is produced from fetal life until puberty. In early puberty, spermatogenesis is initiated by FSH through Sertoli cell proliferation and a subsequent rise in testosterone levels. As a result, the first sign of puberty is an increase in testicular volume with Sertoli cells accounting for 93%–95% of the testicular mass [43].

As Sertoli cells mature, inhibin B and testosterone levels rise, while MIS levels decrease. Inhibin B is germ cell dependent in post pubertal boys and as such is a sensitive marker for germ cell damage in adults [43]; whereas MIS can be used as a marker of Sertoli cell function.

Recent studies suggest that delayed puberty and infertility in NS males may be the result of Sertoli and Leydig cell dysfunction [12]. Marcus et al., studying nine male NS patients, showed Sertoli cells dysfunction by demonstrating decreased levels of inhibin B. In the same study, one-third of patients had normal testicular descent [7]. This is also supported by observations of delayed puberty and impaired fertility in NS males without cryptorchidism [10, 43].

In a longitudinal study by Ankarberg-Lindgren et al., the authors found that over 80% of males with NS had lower testicular volumes than controls during pubertal development. However, as adults, testicular volumes normalized in a majority of these patients [43]. Prepubertal and pubertal levels of testosterone, inhibin B, and MIS in NS patients with and without cryptorchidism were all normal. During puberty, LH levels are elevated in NS patients with cryptorchidism [11], while those without cryptorchidism had normal LH levels [43]. Similarly, FSH levels were found to be increased in NS patients with cryptorchidism during puberty compared to controls. Both inhibin B and MIS levels were lower in NS patients irrespective of cryptorchid status. As adults, NS males with and without cryptorchidism had higher FSH and testosterone levels than controls, whereas MIS and inhibin B levels were lower [44].

These findings prompted Ankarberg-Lindgren et al. to conclude that delayed puberty based on testicular volume may not be an accurate assessment tool to classify pubertal maturation. They postulated that the lower testicular volume is secondary to impaired Sertoli proliferation. Instead, they suggest measuring hormonal levels in NS patients to determine pubertal stage.

Fertility is commonly impaired in males with NS. Impaired spermatogenesis occurs in 60%–80% of NS males [7, 11, 45]. Semen analysis of infertile NS males shows either azoospermia or severe oligozoospermia [44, 45]. Conversely, fertility is preserved in NS females, despite delayed menarche [43]. Sexual dysfunction has not been reported in patients with NS.

Cryptorchidism is currently considered the foremost cause of impaired fertility in NS males. Elsawi et al. studying 11 adult NS patients showed that only 1 out of 9 patients with cryptorchidism fathered children [44]. In addition, this association between cryptorchidism and fertility is well recognized in the adult literature [45, 46]. Azoospermia is found in 89% of men with untreated bilateral cryptorchidism [47]. However, the lower MIS and inhibin B levels in adults with NS indicate progressive Sertoli cell impairment, which may also contribute to impaired spermatogenesis and infertility.

Management

The management of infertility in NS patients should be deferred to an infertility specialist and approached without much deviation from standard infertility evaluation as indicated by international societies. These include the American Urological Association (AUA), the Canadian Urological Association (CUA), and the European Urological Association (EUA). The management algorithm for an infertile NS patient is summarized in Fig. 8.

Unique aspects of infertility care and management for NS patients include the high likelihood of some degree of Sertoli cell dysfunction, or testicular dysgenesis either as a primary dysfunction or secondary to cryptorchidism. Nonobstructive azoospermia and oligozoospermia are the most common presentations. Semen analysis is abnormal in 33%–66% of NS patients, but data on this is severely limited to case series [44]. Interestingly, hormonal abnormalities described in NS men demonstrate normal LH, but elevated FSH in 75%. This supports the idea of intrinsic Sertoli cell dysfunction, but not of classic primary testicular failure given the normal levels of LH and testosterone [7].

Initial evaluation of the infertile NS patient should follow standard guidelines. The standard definition of 12 months of sexual activity without conception still applies as some NS patients are able to father children without medical assistance. A full history and physical examination is required to

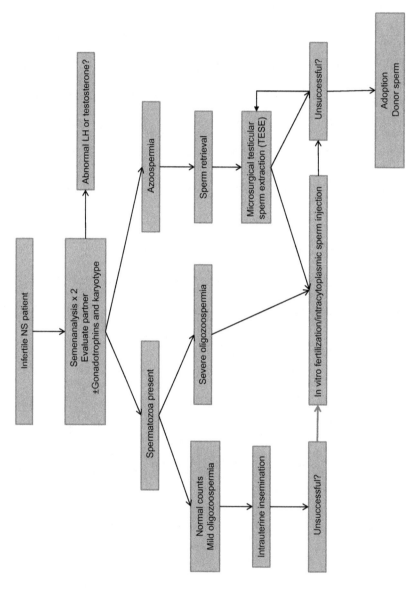

Fig. 8 The management algorithm of an infertile NS male.

identify other risk factors that may alter management. Investigations should include a pair of semen analyses separated by at least a month with 2–5 days of antecedent abstinence.

In NS patients, an argument can be made for early testing of serum gonadotrophins as there is a high rate of abnormalities identified in the literature. In the context of abnormal gonadotrophins, atrophic testicles on physical examination, previous history of cryptorchidism and/or severe oligozoospermia or azoospermia, the discussion toward advanced reproductive techniques should be entered early with NS patients. Additionally, a conversation on genetic counseling should be entertained as discussed previously.

Oligozoospermia Initial semen analysis parameters should include advanced testing such as total motile count, % normal forms, viability, teratospermic index, round cells, microscopy and motility. Assuming the female partner has been thoroughly investigated and found to have no significant abnormalities contributing to infertility, the couple should be approached as a standard infertile couple. Depending on the number of healthy spermatozoa found and their quality, different advanced reproductive technological options can be considered.

In a study by Okuyama et al., seven patients with NS and bilateral cryptorchidism, aged 5–16 years old, were endocrinologically evaluated with LH-RH and HCG stimulation tests, as well as long-term HCG stimulation test and testicular biopsies [48]. Histological examination of the tests confirmed interstitial fibrosis in every case and demonstrated abnormalities of the seminiferous tubules in four patients, while in one patient the seminiferous tubules showed the presence of spermatocytes and spermatids. Similarly, Sasagawa et al. studied the testicular histology and gonadal function of two patients with NS and bilateral cryptorchidism. The authors found elevated plasma FSH levels, but plasma levels of LH, prolactin, and testosterone were within normal ranges in both cases. The administration of LH-RH resulted in an abnormally high response of plasma gonadotropins in both cases. The response of plasma testosterone to the administration of LH-RH was poor in one patient, while normal in the other. Histological examination of the testicles showed reduction of tubular diameter, Leydig cells per seminiferous tubules, and spermatogonia per tubule in both cases. The results indicate an abnormal hypothalamo-pituitary-gonadal axis in NS patients with bilateral cryptorchism [49].

A case report by Kauschansky et al. of a 13-year-old prepubertal boy with NS illustrates the difficulty of predicting potential fertility. The patient had normal basal LH (0.8 mIU/mL) levels, while the FSH level (2.5 mIU/mL) was high. Both LH and FSH (8.3 mIU/mL and 9.6 mIU/mL, respectively) showed an elevated response to LH-RH, which is normally seen in primary hypogonadism. However, the patient had a normal testosterone response to HCG (437 ng%) [50].

Individual fertility centers will have their own protocols, however good quality semen may be a candidate for intrauterine insemination, and poor quality or very few sperm may be directed toward in vitro fertilization/intracytoplasmic sperm injection (IVF/ICSI). The main advantage of course is that the ability to collect spermatozoa is considerably easier and less morbid than those with nonobstructive azoospermia. If there are continued issues with fertility after several rounds of IVF/ICSI, it may then be a consideration to discuss donor sperm or adoption.

Azoospermia Standard evaluation of nonobstructive azoospermia should be performed. Karyotype and Y microdeletion tests are warranted in patients with nonobstructive azoospermia [51]. If not performed already, gonadotrophins should be ordered and reviewed. Typical patterns for NS patients include normal testosterone and LH, with abnormal FSH levels in isolation. This would not be a typical picture for primary testicular failure, or secondary testicular failure from pituitary dysfunction. There is no evidence that any hormonal manipulation may improve sperm production in NS patients.

Aspiration techniques have low morbidity but are unlikely to be successful in the azoospermic NS patient based on our current understanding of the pathophysiology but may be attempted at the same time of microsurgical approaches. Microsurgical dissection techniques allow an opportunity for the azoospermic patient to sire children, and in the azoospermic NS patient this may be the only option for paternity.

These procedures are typically followed with IVF/ICSI and individual fertility centers will report their own sperm retrieval and pregnancy rates. Data from Cornell however has been reported to have rates of 64% and 50% in sperm retrieval and pregnancy in patients with a previous history of cryptorchidism and azoospermia [52, 53]. Interestingly, focal spermatogenesis appears to be present in those previously labeled as Sertoli cell only, and sperm retrieval rates of 44% have been reported from the same group with subsequent pregnancy rates of approximately 46% [34].

No data specific to microsurgical dissection techniques and subsequent pregnancy rates have been reported in NS patients, and therefore these numbers must be discussed with NS couples with caution. If sperm retrieval is unsuccessful, repeat attempts can be made but typically with diminishing returns of success. At some point, an honest and open discussion regarding donor sperm and adoption must be entered into, however exactly when that should happen is not clear.

ONCOLOGICAL TUMORS

Children with NS have an increased risk for developing both benign and malignant proliferative disorders. Mild myeloproliferative disorders affect approximately 10% of children with NS. NS is also associated with an increased risk for juvenile myelomonocytic leukemia and other hematological malignancies. In one-third of children with these hematological cancers, a somatic missense mutation in *PTPN11* is found [4]. However, there has been no conclusive evidence a causative role of *PTPN11* in the development of these malignancies.

Children with NS have also been associated with certain solid tumors such as neuroblastoma, embryonal rhabdomyosarcoma, and giant cell tumors of the jaw [54]. Denayer et al. found malignancies in 3 out of 10 patients with SOS1 mutations including one with embryonal rhabdomyosarcoma originating from the urachus. The SOS1 germline mutation has also been reported in NS patients with Sertoli cell tumors [8].

Children with NS who are *PTPN11* positive have a cumulative cancer risk of 23%, which is a 3.5-fold increased risk compared to the general population [4]. Although to date there is no conclusive evidence on the influence of *PTPN11* on the development of malignancies. Tumor surveillance is often difficult, in part due to variability in site of these malignancies and the differences in age of presentation. As such, the development of an effective screening protocol is difficult for NS patients.

Management

The management of oncological tumors in NS patients should be referred to a pediatric oncologist. From a urological prospective, the incidence of genitourinary relevant tumors is exceedingly rare. The specific management of neuroblastoma and embryonal rhabdomyosarcoma pertaining to urology is exhaustive and beyond the scope of this chapter. Briefly, the patient should be evaluated, and a tissue diagnosis should be obtained that will further guide staging and management.

REFERENCES

[1] Noonan JA. Hypertelorism with Turner phenotype. A new syndrome with associated congenital heart disease. Am J Dis Child 1968;116(4):373–80.

[2] Heller RH. The Turner phenotype in the male. J Pediatr 1965;66:48–63.

[3] Romano AA, et al. Noonan syndrome: clinical features, diagnosis, and management guidelines. Pediatrics 2010;126(4):746–59.

[4] Jongmans MC, et al. Cancer risk in patients with Noonan syndrome carrying a PTPN11 mutation. Eur J Hum Genet 2011;19(8):870–4.

[5] Jongmans M, et al. Genetics and variation in phenotype in Noonan syndrome. Horm Res 2004;62(Suppl. 3):56–9.

[6] Brady AF, et al. Further delineation of the critical region for Noonan syndrome on the long arm of chromosome 12. Eur J Hum Genet 1997;5(5):336–7.

[7] Marcus KA, et al. Impaired Sertoli cell function in males diagnosed with Noonan syndrome. J Pediatr Endocrinol Metab 2008;21(11):1079–84.

[8] Roberts AE, et al. Noonan syndrome. Lancet 2013;381(9863):333–42.

[9] Digilio M, Marino B. Clinical manifestations of Noonan syndrome. Images Paediatr Cardiol 2001;3(2):19–30.

[10] Bhambhani V, Muenke M. Noonan syndrome. Am Fam Physician 2014;89(1):37–43.

[11] Theintz G, Savage MO. Growth and pubertal development in five boys with Noonan's syndrome. Arch Dis Child 1982;57(1):13–7.

[12] Chacko E, et al. Update on Turner and Noonan syndromes. Endocrinol Metab Clin N Am 2012;41(4):713–34.

[13] Myers A, et al. Perinatal features of the RASopathies: Noonan syndrome, cardiofacio-cutaneous syndrome and Costello syndrome. Am J Med Genet A 2014;164A (11):2814–21.

[14] George CD, et al. Abdominal ultrasound in Noonan syndrome: a study of 44 patients. Pediatr Radiol 1993;23(4):316–8.

[15] Raghavaiah NV. Noonan's syndrome associated with cake kidney. Urology 1975;5 (5):640–2.

[16] Gupta A, et al. Noonan syndrome: crossed fused ectopic kidneys and focal segmental glomerulosclerosis—a rare association. Clin Exp Nephrol 2009;13(5):531–2.

[17] Semizel E, Bostan OM, Saglam H. Bilateral multiple pulmonary arteriovenous fistulas and duplicated renal collecting system in a child with Noonan's syndrome. Cardiol Young 2007;17(2):229–31.

[18] Barker M, Engelhardt W. Bilateral kidney duplication in familial Noonan's syndrome. Clin Pediatr (Phila) 2001;40(4):241–2.

[19] Tejani A, et al. Noonan's syndrome associated with polycystic renal disease. J Urol 1976;115(2):209–11.

[20] Hellebusch AA. Noonan syndrome with bilateral ureteral ectopia. J Pediatr Surg 1971;6 (4):490.

[21] Hutson JM, et al. The regulation of testicular descent and the effects of cryptorchidism. Endocr Rev 2013;34(5):725–52.

[22] Sharland M, et al. A clinical study of Noonan syndrome. Arch Dis Child 1992;67 (2):178–83.

[23] Diemer T, Desjardins C. Developmental and genetic disorders in spermatogenesis. Hum Reprod Update 1999;5(2):120–40.

[24] Hutson JM, Hasthorpe S. Testicular descent and cryptorchidism: the state of the art in 2004. J Pediatr Surg 2005;40(2):297–302.

[25] Zimmermann S, et al. Targeted disruption of the Insl3 gene causes bilateral cryptorchidism. Mol Endocrinol 1999;13(5):681–91.

[26] Kaftanovskaya EM, et al. Cryptorchidism in mice with an androgen receptor ablation in gubernaculum testis. Mol Endocrinol 2012;26(4):598–607.

[27] Sampaio FJ, Favorito LA. Analysis of testicular migration during the fetal period in humans. J Urol 1998;159(2):540–2.

[28] Chan JJ, et al. Calcitonin gene-related peptide is a survival factor, inhibiting apoptosis in neonatal rat gubernaculum in vitro. J Pediatr Surg 2009;44(8):1497–501.

[29] Niikura H, et al. Fetal development of the human gubernaculum with special reference to the fasciae and muscles around it. Clin Anat 2008;21(6):547–57.

[30] Lindsey S, et al. Activation of SHP2 protein-tyrosine phosphatase increases HoxA10-induced repression of the genes encoding gp91(PHOX) and p67(PHOX). J Biol Chem 2007;282(4):2237–49.

[31] Rijli FM, et al. Cryptorchidism and homeotic transformations of spinal nerves and vertebrae in Hoxa-10 mutant mice. Proc Natl Acad Sci U S A 1995;92(18):8185–9.

[32] Kolon TF, et al. Evaluation and treatment of cryptorchidism: AUA guideline. J Urol 2014;192(2):337–45.

[33] Ritzen EM. Undescended testes: a consensus on management. Eur J Endocrinol 2008;159(Suppl. 1):S87–90.

[34] Chung E, Brock GB. Cryptorchidism and its impact on male fertility: a state of art review of current literature. Can Urol Assoc J 2011;5(3):210–4.

[35] Wagner-Mahler K, et al. Prospective study on the prevalence and associated risk factors of cryptorchidism in 6246 newborn boys from Nice area, France. Int J Androl 2011;34 (5 Pt 2):e499–510.

[36] Wenzler DL, Bloom DA, Park JM. What is the rate of spontaneous testicular descent in infants with cryptorchidism? J Urol 2004;171(2 Pt 1):849–51.

[37] Kollin C, et al. Testicular growth from birth to two years of age, and the effect of orchidopexy at age nine months: a randomized, controlled study. Acta Paediatr 2006;95 (3):318–24.

[38] Peters CA. Laparoscopy in pediatric urology. Curr Opin Urol 2004;14(2):67–73.

[39] Hinman FJ. Testis: repair and reconstruction. In: Atlas of urologic surgery. Philadelphia, PA: W.B. Saunders Company; 1998. p. 308–15.

[40] Orlando R, Palatini P, Lirussi F. Needle and trocar injuries in diagnostic laparoscopy under local anesthesia: what is the true incidence of these complications? J Laparoendosc Adv Surg Tech A 2003;13(3):181–4.

[41] Pastor N, et al. Noonan syndrome and scrotal lymphedema: primary or secondary? Pediatr Dermatol 2006;23(4):411–2.

[42] Nistal M, Paniagua R, Bravo MP. Testicular lymphangiectasis in Noonan's syndrome. J Urol 1984;131(4):759–61.

[43] Ankarberg-Lindgren C, Westphal O, Dahlgren J. Testicular size development and reproductive hormones in boys and adult males with Noonan syndrome: a longitudinal study. Eur J Endocrinol 2011;165(1):137–44.

[44] Elsawi MM, et al. Genital tract function in men with Noonan syndrome. J Med Genet 1994;31(6):468–70.

[45] Sinisi AA, et al. Endocrine profile in Noonan's syndrome. Minerva Endocrinol 1987;12 (1):13–7.

[46] Huff DS, et al. Abnormal germ cell development in cryptorchidism. Horm Res 2001;55 (1):11–7.

[47] Hadziselimovic F, Herzog B. The importance of both an early orchidopexy and germ cell maturation for fertility. Lancet 2001;358(9288):1156–7.

[48] Okuyama A, et al. Gonadal findings in cryptorchid boys with Noonan's phenotype. Eur Urol 1981;7(5):274–7.

[49] Sasagawa I, et al. Gonadal function and testicular histology in Noonan's syndrome with bilateral cryptorchidism. Arch Androl 1994;32(2):135–40.

[50] Kauschansky A, Eilam N, Elian E. LH-RH and HCG studies in a Turner phenotype male (Noonan's syndrome). A case report. Helv Paediat Acta 1977;32(3):237–40.

[51] Gangel EK, American Urological Association, Inc, American Society for Reproductive Medicine. AUA and ASRM produce recommendations for male infertility. American Urological Association, Inc and American Society for Reproductive Medicine. Am Fam Physician 2002;65(12):2589–90.
[52] Su LM, et al. Testicular sperm extraction with intracytoplasmic sperm injection for non-obstructive azoospermia: testicular histology can predict success of sperm retrieval. J Urol 1999;161(1):112–6.
[53] Schlegel PN. Testicular sperm extraction: microdissection improves sperm yield with minimal tissue excision. Hum Reprod 1999;14(1):131–5.
[54] Denayer E, et al. Tumor spectrum in children with Noonan syndrome and SOS1 or RAF1 mutations. Genes Chromosom Cancer 2010;49(3):242–52.

CHAPTER 6

Gastrointestinal Manifestations of Noonan Syndrome

Rishi Gupta*, Ashish Chogle[†]
*Division of Pediatric Gastroenterology, University of Maryland Medical Center, Baltimore, MD, United States
†Division of Pediatric Gastroenterology, Children's Hospital of Orange County, Orange, CA, United States

Abbreviations

CFCS   cardio-facio-cutaneous syndrome
CS   Costello syndrome
ERK   extracellular signal-regulated kinases
JAK   Janus kinase
MAPK   mitogen-activated protein kinase
NS   Noonan syndrome
STAT   signal transducer of activation

Abstract

A large percentage of children with Noonan syndrome experience feeding difficulties due to oro-motor deficits, malocclusion, gastroesophageal reflux, and possible upper gastrointestinal dysmotility. Appropriate intervention by physical and occupational therapy can improve oral intake. Some children also need enteral feedings to support their nutritional needs. With advancing age, lot of these children have improved feeding tolerance and less dependence on enteral nutrition.

Keywords: Gastroesophageal reflux, Gastroduodenal motility, Dental malformations, Noonan syndrome, Nutrition, Malformations, Feeding difficulty

INTRODUCTION

Noonan syndrome (NS) is an autosomal dominant disorder characterized by short stature, facial dysmorphism (downslanting palpebral fissures, proptosis, ocular hypertelorism, palpebral ptosis, dental malocclusion, and overfolded pinnae), sternal deformities, short and/or webbed neck, congenital heart disease, bleeding diathesis, and cryptorchidism [1]. Mutations in several genes acting in the RAS/MAPK (mitogen-activated protein kinase) pathway result in the phenotype of NS as well as other rare syndromes with characteristics similar to NS. The Noonan-related disorders include cardio-facio-cutaneous syndrome (CFCS), Noonan syndrome with multiple lentigines (NSML) or LEOPARD syndrome, Noonan-like syndrome Legius

Noonan Syndrome
https://doi.org/10.1016/B978-0-12-815348-2.00005-0

syndrome (NSLS), neurofibromatosis type 1 (NF1), Noonan-like syndrome with loose anagen hair (NSLAH) and Costello syndrome (CS). These disorders represent a group of genetic conditions collectively also known as RASopathies [1,2]. The RASopathies represent one of the most prevalent groups of developmental malformation syndromes, affecting more than 1 in 1000 individuals [3]. Each RASopathy is a distinct syndrome caused by mutations at different points in the pathway, and these syndromes share many overlapping characteristics, including craniofacial malformations, musculoskeletal anomalies, cutaneous lesions, cardiovascular abnormalities, neurocognitive impairment, and increased risk of tumor formation [2].

There is very limited data available in literature, regarding gastrointestinal issues in patients with NS or other RASopathies. In clinical practice, a large majority of infants with NS encounter feeding difficulties. The mechanisms that could lead to feeding difficulties in infants with NS are manifold such as dental and mandibular malformations, gastroesophageal reflux disease or GERD, abnormal gastro-duodenal motility and increased incidence of gastrointestinal structural anomalies such as midgut malrotation and hiatal hernia.

NUTRITION IN NS PATIENTS

Growth impairment is a hallmark of RASopathies, which is present in 50%–60% of individuals with NS, which is by far the most prevalent syndrome among the various RASopathies. Growth impairment is characterized as proportionate and of postnatal origin [4]. Birth weight is usually normal in NS and may even be increased due to edema.

Infants with NS can then present with failure to thrive caused by feeding difficulties such as poor suck, prolonged feeding times, and recurrent vomiting [5,6]. A large retrospective study of infants with NS found 76% infants with varying degrees of feeding difficulty. Of these patients, 15% of children have been reported with mild feeding difficulty, which is defined as poor suck with prolonged feeding time lasting over an hour during infancy; 38% had moderate feeding difficulty which is very poor suck, with slow feeding and recurrent vomiting with most feeds; and 24% of the children had a severe feeding problems, requiring tube feedings for 2 weeks or longer in a term infant [5]. Similar feeding difficulties that have been associated with RASopathies, especially in CS and CFCS, which tend to show a pronounced phenotype of failure to thrive [5,7,8]. Although these feeding difficulties usually resolve in the first few years of life, lower BMI values are reported in children with NS and other RASopathies and are correlated with a lower prevalence of overweight and obesity in adults when compared with the general population [4, 9–12]. As the daily energy and nutrient intake seem to be normal in NS children, their lower BMI may be related to increased energy expenditure [4]. Similarly, patients with CS also display increased energy expenditure despite normal daily caloric intake [10]. Recent studies have shown that dysregulation of RAS/MAPK pathway could play a role in metabolism and energy storage, as demonstrated by the low BMI in RASopathy patients and lean habitus in transgenic knock-in mice [11]. Moreover, mice expressing an NSML *Ptpn11* gene loss-of-function mutation as opposed to gain-of-function mutation seen in NS presents in a similar manner of increased energy expenditure, secondary to enhanced mitochondria biogenesis/activity [13]. These effects involved signaling molecules ERK 1/2, JAK2, and STAT3. However, the exact metabolic mechanism of the MAPK/ERK pathway, lower BMI, and the lower prevalence of obesity in NS are not fully understood [12].

CRANIOFACIAL AND DENTAL MANIFESTATIONS IN NS PATIENTS

In the review of oral manifestations in patients with NS, a number of facial and dental anomalies have been reported to occur such as of malocclusion, high arch palate, micrognathia, enamel hypoplasia leading to feeding difficulties, labial hypotonia, gingival inflammation, proclined incisors, and supernumerary teeth [14]. The distribution of these anomalies in NS patients is not uniform, and these may or may not be associated with the general manifestations of NS, including cardiac and other anomalies. The oral lesions may lead to feeding difficulties due to poor suck, poor latching to breast and bottle during infancy, and poor mastication, after teeth have erupted. It has been recommended that patients with NS should be screened for oral health in the first year of life to prevent and treat these issues. It is also important to continuously monitor the oral health of these patients, as they are prone to developing gingival problems, dental caries and issues with eruption of permanent teeth, leading to feeding problems. (For more detailed discussion regarding dental malformations, please refer to Chapter 10.)

FOREGUT DYSMOTILITY IN NS PATIENTS

The role of foregut dysmotility in the causation of feeding difficulties has also been demonstrated in infants and children with NS [7]. In this study, poor feeding was defined as poor suck, refusal to eat or drink, and recurrent vomiting, which was noted to be present in 64% patients. All these patients required tube feedings due to severe feeding difficulties. Of these children, 12% had midgut malrotation, 31% had hiatal hernia, and 44% had gastro-esophageal reflux as diagnosed by 24-h pH probe monitoring. Gastroesoph-ageal reflux can predispose to esophagitis and silent aspiration leading to secondary feeding problems. Five children in this cohort underwent electro-gastrography and four were found to have abnormal gastric myo-electric activity, which authors postulated to be linked to delayed gastric emptying. Four children had antro-duodenal manometry and were found to have abnormal studies. The myoelectric activity recorded was similar to that seen in premature infants of 32–35 weeks gestational age. In most of the patients included in this study, the feeding problem improved with age. This study supported the theory that the delayed development of central nervous system in NS parallels delayed development of autonomic enteric nervous system, which governs the stomach and intestine myoelectric activity [7].

In another study of 116 infants with NS, the correlation of feeding prob-lems was observed with other delays in development and with the need for special education. Based on these findings, they postulated that feeding problem in infancy could be a neonatal marker for poorer long-term devel-opmental outcome in patients with NS [6].

EVALUATION FOR FEEDING DIFFICULTIES IN A CHILD

Feeding evaluation in a child irrespective of any underlying organic disease is a comprehensive undertaking. It starts with taking detailed feeding history from care providers and observing feeding or meal session of a child in a non-interventionist way. Child might need further evaluation from a dental sur-geon, ENT surgeon, gastroenterologist, and speech and occupational therapist as needed based on initial assessment. Most children need an eso-phagogram or an upper gastrointestinal series. These are radiological tests to evaluate for structural pharyngeal and gastroesophageal abnormalities and intestinal malrotation. They also need a video fluoroscopic swallow study (VFSS) or fiberoptic endoscopic evaluation of swallowing (FEES) to assess oropharyngeal swallow function. Another useful tool is 24-h esophageal pH probe along with impedance measurement. This test evaluates for the pres-ence of gastroesophageal reflux, both acidic and nonacidic reflux events. Electro-gastrography studies are not used much these days due to lack of correlation between patient's symptoms and study results. Similarly, gastric emptying study using liquid diets is not very informative for gastric emptying function. This study might be more useful in children who can ingest a solid meal. Occasionally an esophagogastroduodenoscopy with biopsies is needed to evaluate for underlying eosinophilic esophagitis (EoE), which is food allergy-related condition leading to esophageal wall thickening, impaired motility, and gradual esophageal stricture formation. EoE is usually seen in patients with other underlying allergic predispositions, such as asthma, seasonal allergies, eczema, and family history of allergies. Still, this condition can be missed if not thought about and leads to progressive difficulty in advancing feeds in a child. Esophageal manometry is not often used in this group of children for feeding difficulty evaluation but an occasional patient might need this study if there are specific symptoms suggesting esophageal dysmotility. A majority of children with organic feeding difficulties in infancy develop secondary feeding aversion. Despite improvement in their oropharyngeal swallow function and gastroesophageal reflux, they have perceived discomfort with feeding. Severe feeding aversion in some children with NS can lead to difficulty in advancing oral feeds and gradual dependence on gastrostomy tube to meet nutritional needs.

MANAGEMENT OF FEEDING DIFFICULTIES AND CORRECTING MALNUTRITION

Identification and treatment for malocclusion of jaw, using appropriate nipple for high arched palate along with palatal prosthesis or surgical repair, can help with infant's sucking ability. Labial and pharyngeal hypotonia can respond to occupational therapy. Infantile gastroesophageal reflux can be managed conservatively by using correct feeding position and thickening of the formula. Occasionally, medications such as H2 receptor blocker, ranitidine, can also be helpful in alleviating the reflux-like symptoms. Erythromycin and metoclopramide are prokinetic medications, which are used in patients with severe gastroesophageal reflux, foregut dysmotility, and delayed gastric emptying. Cyproheptadine is another medication which is used as an appetite stimulant and to increase the gastric accommodation. Primary and secondary feeding aversions need behavioral feeding therapy through a feeding team in collaboration with parents.

CONCLUSION

In conclusion, early onset feeding difficulties are common in children with NS. Infants with NS and other similar RASopathies are at higher risk of developing feeding issues secondary to oro-dento-facial abnormalities and along with gut motility issues due to the delayed development of autonomic enteric nervous system. NS children with feeding difficulties need an early assessment and a team approach to proper evaluation and management of feeding difficulties. A systematic approach in arriving at a correct diagnosis for feeding disorder and providing appropriate treatment goes a long way in making these children nutritionally sufficient and independent from enteral nutrition.

CONFLICT OF INTEREST

None to declare.

REFERENCES

[1] Romano AA, Allanson JE, Dahlgren J, Gelb BD, Hall B, Pierpont ME, et al. Noonan syndrome: clinical features, diagnosis, and management guidelines. Pediatrics 2010;126 (4):746–59.

[2] Rauen KA. The RASopathies. Annu Rev Genomics Hum Genet 2013;14:355–69.

[3] Tidyman WE, Rauen KA. Pathogenetics of the RASopathies. Hum Mol Genet 2016;25(R2):R123–32.

[4] da Silva FM, Jorge AA, Malaquias A, da Costa PA, Yamamoto GL, Kim CA, et al. Nutritional aspects of Noonan syndrome and Noonan-related disorders. Am J Med Genet A 2016;170(6):1525–31.

[5] Sharland M, Burch M, McKenna WM, Paton MA. A clinical study of Noonan syndrome. Arch Dis Child 1992;67(2):178–83.

[6] Shaw AC, Kalidas K, Crosby AH, Jeffery S, Patton MA. The natural history of Noonan syndrome: a long-term follow-up study. Arch Dis Child 2007;92(2):128–32. https:// doi.org/10.1136/adc.2006.104547 [Epub 2006 Sep 21].

[7] Shah N, Rodriguez M, Louis DS, Lindley K, Milla PJ. Feeding difficulties and foregut dysmotility in Noonan's syndrome. Arch Dis Child 1999;81(1):28–31.

[8] Gripp KW, Zand DJ, Demmer L, Anderson CE, Dobyns WB, Zackai EH, et al. Expanding the SHOC2 mutation associated phenotype of Noonan syndrome with loose anagen hair: structural brain anomalies and myelofibrosis. Am J Med Genet A 2013;161A(10):2420–30.

[9] Cessans C, Ehlinger V, Arnaud C, Yart A, Capri Y, Barat P, et al. Growth patterns of patients with Noonan syndrome: correlation with age and genotype. Eur J Endocrinol 2016;174(5):641–50.

[10] Leoni C, Onesimo R, Giorgio V, Diamanti A, Giorgio D, Martini L, et al. Understanding growth failure in Costello syndrome: increased resting energy expenditure. J Pediatr 2016;170:322–4.

[11] Malaquias AC, Brasil AS, Pereira AC, Arnhold IJ, Mendonca BB, Bertola DR, et al. Growth standards of patients with Noonan and Noonan-like syndromes with mutations in the RAS/MAPK pathway. Am J Med Genet A 2012;158A(11):2700–6.

[12] Binder G, Grathwol S, von Loeper K, Blumenstock G, Kaulitz R, Freiberg C, et al. Health and quality of life in adults with Noonan syndrome. J Pediatr 2012;161 (3):501–505.e1.

[13] Tajan M, Batut A, Cadoudal T, Deleruyelle S, Le Gonidec S, Saint Laurent C, et al. LEOPARD syndrome-associated SHP2 mutation confers leanness and protection from diet-induced obesity. Proc Natl Acad Sci U S A 2014;111(42):E4494–503.

[14] Mallineni SK, Yung Yiu CK, King NM. Oral manifestations of Noonan syndrome: review of the literature and a report of four cases. Rom J Morphol Embryol 2014;55 (4):1503–9.

CHAPTER 7

Developmental and Neurological Features of Noonan Syndrome

Minodora O. Totoiu
Division of Pediatric Neurology, Children's Hospital Orange County, University of California Irvine Medical Center, Orange, CA, United States

Abstract

The neurological aspects, including cognitive and behavioral functioning, of the clinical manifestations of individuals with Noonan syndrome (NS) are extremely variable and poorly understood. Results of different studies have yielded variable data, but showed that a large proportion of the patients with NS were affected in different areas of the nervous system: central nervous system malformations, cerebrovascular abnormalities, developmental delays, speech disorders, early motor milestones delay, hypotonia and hypermobility of joints, recurrent seizures, ocular problems, hearing loss and neuromuscular (peripheral neuropathy). Although most individuals with NS have normal intelligence, about one third have a mild intellectual disability, some have learning difficulties and psychological and behavioral problems, such as stubbornness, irritability, and poor self-esteem. This variability is likely related to the patient's specific genetic mutation.

Keywords: Neurological manifestations, Developmental milestones, Cognition, Speech/language, Learning, Behavior, Psychological and mental health

Nomenclature

ADHD	Attention Deficit Hyperactivity Disorder
ASD	autism spectrum disorder
EEG	Electroencephalography
FS-IQ	full-scale intelligence quotient
GABA	gamma aminobutyric acid
GTPase	Guanosine Triphosphatase
IQ	intelligence quotient
MAPK – RAS	mitogen activated protein kinase signaling pathway
MAPK/ERK	mitogen activated protein kinase signaling cascade
MCHAT	Modified Checklist for Autism in Toddlers
MRI	magnetic resonance Imaging
NS	Noonan syndrome
WRAML-2	Wide Range Assessment of Memory and Learning, Second Edition

Noonan Syndrome
https://doi.org/10.1016/B978-0-12-815348-2.00006-2

INTRODUCTION

Noonan syndrome (NS) is an autosomal dominant multisystem disorder variably expressed. Affected individuals have distinctive facial features, short stature, cardiovascular defects, and other congenital anomalies [1]. The estimated prevalence of NS is between 1:1000 and 1:2500 live births [2]. Most physicians will treat patients with NS during their career. NS is caused by the dysregulation and/or mutations in genes in the RAS-mitogen activated protein kinase (MAPK) signaling pathway (Fig. 1). This pathway is essential in the regulation of the cell differentiation, growth, and senescence, all of

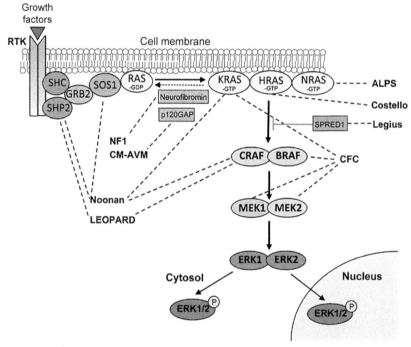

Fig. 1 The Ras/mitogen-activated protein kinase (MAPK) signaling pathway and associated developmental syndromes (indicated by *dashed lines*). The MAPK signaling pathway of protein kinases is critically involved in cell proliferation, differentiation, motility, apoptosis and senescence. The Ras/MAPK pathway proteins with germline mutations in their respective genes are associated with Noonan, LEOPARD, gingival fibromatosis 1, neurofibromatosis 1, capillary malformation-arteriovenous malformation, Costello, autoimmune lymphoproliferative (ALPS), cardio-facio-cutaneous and Legius syndromes. *(Permission pending Tidyman WE, Rauen KA. The RASopathies: developmental syndromes of Ras/MAPK pathway dysregulation. Curr Opin Genet Dev. 2009;19(3):230–6.)*

which are critical to normal development [3,4]. NS has high phenotypic variability and shares clinical features with other rare conditions from the group of so-called RASopathies. These include LEOPARD syndrome, craniofaciocutaneous syndrome, Costello syndrome, and Noonan-like syndrome with loose anagen hair [5]. Besides the common manifestations (cardiac disease, short stature, and facial anomalies), in certain patients, the syndrome has developmental and neurological implications.

Noonan syndrome was first described by pediatric cardiologist Dr. Jacqueline Noonan in 1963. Heterogenous clinical findings, including developmental and neurological conditions, were observed. Most patients have a normal intelligence quotient (IQ) but up to 35% may have mild intellectual disability. Some affected individuals may have abnormal delays of skills requiring the coordination of mental and muscular activity, learning disabilities, and language delays. These delays may manifest as hypotonia, difficulties in speaking, mild hearing loss. Inattention and challenges with executive functioning have also been reported. Many adults have relatively normal cognitive functioning except for lower information processing speed [6].

MOLECULAR PATHOGENESIS

Noonan syndrome is part of the group of so-called RASopathies, which are caused by mutations in the genes that encode for the ERK-MAP kinase signaling pathway. These mutations have profound effects on cellular development. The ERK-MAPK pathway is downstream from the fibroblast growth factor receptor. Disruption of the ERK-MAPK pathway during embryogenesis impedes neural crest cell development and causes defects in cardiac, craniofacial, and central nervous system structures [7].

The MAPK/ERK pathway (Ras-Raf-MEK-ERK pathway) consists of a series of intracellular proteins which facilitate the transmission of information from extracellular receptors to the nuclear DNA and other cytoplasmic effectors. This pathway regulates the activity of transcription factors. Cellular growth and differentiation are controlled by multiple extracellular signals, many of which activate this pathway (the Ras/mitogen-activated protein (MAP or ERK) kinase cascade). These extracellular signals, regulated by the kinase (ERK) subfamily of mitogen-activated protein (MAP) kinases, comprise the central elements of one of the most important and best-studied intracellular signaling pathways [8]. These receptors are physically and functionally linked to the ERK cascade through a diverse group of molecular adapters that couple them to the activation of the GTPases of the Ras family. The MAPK/ERK signaling cascade plays an important/critical role in brain development, memory, learning, and cognition. Mutations in this pathway can cause developmental syndromes [7]. RAS proteins activated via phosphorylation events will activate the RAF-MEK-ERK cascade. The activated ERK enters the nucleus and will modulate transcription and activity of cytoplasmic targets. These effects will generate short-term and long-term cellular responses. All the genes implicated in NS code for proteins in this pathway. Abnormal Ras-ERK signaling has also been linked to some neuropsychiatric conditions, mental retardation syndromes, and drug addiction.

During development, the ERKs respond to growth factors through the activation of receptor tyrosine kinases. In the mature nervous system, ERK is part of the mechanism for synaptic plasticity in several different brain structures, and its activation is necessary for the long-term consolidation of memory [9].

During postnatal life the ERK-MAPK pathway is involved in synaptic function, especially in GABAergic neurons. Disruption of GABAergic projections, from the medium spiny neurons in the striatum, interrupts inhibition of excitatory glutamatergic and dopaminergic pathways, leading to cortical inhibitory-excitatory imbalances. Changes in GABAergic function in the hippocampus may affect memory and learning. Mutations or deletions in this signaling pathway generate these imbalances that may lead to developmental syndromes associated with impairment in cognitive functioning and autistic features [10].

The understanding of the role of the RAS-MAPK pathway in neurodevelopment is even more intricate because both loss-of-function and gain-of-function mutations are associated with RASopathies and have been shown to have differential effects on brain function in animal models [11].

DEVELOPMENTAL AND NEUROLOGICAL MANIFESTATIONS

Noonan syndrome is clinically heterogenous, and patients can have different developmental and neurological manifestations, such as early motor milestone delay, hypotonia and joint laxity/hypermobility, central nervous system malformations, learning difficulties, speech/language disorders and behavioral conditions (stubbornness, irritability, body image problems, and poor self-esteem).

BIRTH PARAMETERS

Prenatal features are nonspecific but include polyhydramnios, hydronephrosis, pleural effusion, edema, cardiac defects, distended jugular lymphatic sacs, cystic hygroma, and increased nuchal translucency [12,13]. During intrauterine life, some fetuses may show relative macrocephaly [14]. Birthweight and head circumference and body length at birth are usually normal [5], but approximately 40% of children fail to thrive in infancy [15,16]. According to a clinical study of NS, most patients had a normal head circumference at birth (the group mean was in the 50th percentile), even though the children were short and underweight. Some children had microcephaly or macrocephaly. Also, about 50% had a height less than the 3rd percentile, and 43% had the weight less than in the 3rd percentile [17].

DEVELOPMENTAL MILESTONES

Many children with NS have delays in their early motor development milestones. This may be related to hypotonia and joint hyperextensibility, and, during early childhood, it could be a result of the congenital heart disease, failure to thrive, and skeletal anomalies [1].

According to a study of 151 children with NS in the United Kingdom, 26% had delays in the mean age of motor milestones. The average age for sitting unsupported was around 10 months (SD 4.5 months), in the group of 126 patients for which this information was available. The age of independent walking was available for 112 cases and had a mean of 21 months (SD 10.2 months) [17].

Children with NS showed a higher rate of clumsiness and poor coordination. Seventy-one percent of NS children between 2 and 19 years, in a UK study of 27 NS children, showed clumsiness [18]. Another study showed that developmental coordination disorder was present in about 50% of school-age children. Gross motor skills were more impaired than fine motor skills, communication, and social skills [19]. Subsequent studies confirmed impaired manual dexterity, which was significantly correlated with verbal and nonverbal intellectual functioning on the Purdue Pegboard Test [20].

Children with NS have delay in their speech development. In the study of 151 children with NS, the age of speaking in simple two-word sentences was known for 102 children and occurred around 31 months (SD 9.6 months) [17]. In the same study, hearing tests were performed on 146 members of the group, and hearing loss was reported in 58 children (40%). In a large majority, this was due to serous otitis media. Nerve deafness, requiring hearing aids, was detected in five children (3%) [17].

SPEECH AND LANGUAGE DEVELOPMENT

Speech and language pathology is common in children and adults with NS. A study of language phenotype showed that language impairments were more frequent than in the general population and were associated with higher risk for reading and spelling difficulties [21]. The average age when first words were spoken was around 15 months [21]; and simple two-word phrases emerged, on average, between 31 and 32 months [17]. In this study, the age of two-word phrases was known for 102 children, and this mean age was 31 months (SD of 9.6 months).

Feeding problems during infancy in NS patients were identified as a predictor of language development. The mean age for speaking two-word phrases was 26 months for those with no feeding difficulties and 39 months for those with feeding difficulties that required nasogastric feeding tubes [22]. The feeding problems present were described as poor suck, swallow, or gagging reflex, recurrent vomiting, food refusal, and intestinal dysmotility [23,24].

Language delay was found in 20% of patients with NS and may be related to mild hearing loss, perceptual motor disabilities, or articulation deficiencies. Articulation abnormalities were common (72%), but patients usually responded well to speech therapy [15]. In a study on 66 children and adolescents, language impairment was significantly correlated with nonverbal cognition, hearing, articulation, phonologic memory, and motor dexterity, but no specific aspect of language was selectively affected in these patients [25].

A study of language abilities and pragmatic skills focused on 17 patients with NS and an age and gender matched control group, found that 76.5% of the children in the NS group were identified with language impairments compared to 2 children (11.8%) in the typically developing group [26].

Problems with language development were found to be linked to subsequently delayed development of academic skills. Reading and spelling skills were strongly correlated with language ability and nonverbal cognitive ability in patients with NS [21]. This study also suggested that social aspects of language are also affected, particularly male participants, but more studies regarding social communication are needed.

OCULAR AND VISUAL FINDINGS

Patients with Noonan syndrome are affected by different anatomical ocular abnormalities, widely spaced eyes, down slanting palpebral fissures, ptosis, and ocular motility problems such as nystagmus, strabismus, and vision abnormalities (refractive errors and amblyopia) [27].

Vision abnormalities were found in 94% of patients with NS [17]. In this study of 145 individuals, vision was tested and found to be abnormal in 80 participants (55%). Of these, 52 patients underwent a full orthoptic and ophthalmological evaluation and strabismus and amblyopia were detected in 33 patients (63%) and 16 patients (31%), respectively. Refractive errors (myopia and hypermetropia) were found in 35 patients (67%). In this cohort, normal eye examinations were found in only three patients (6%). In another study, refractive errors were found in 39 of 69 patients (71%), 53% had myopia, 14% had hypermetropia, and 13% had astigmatism. No relationship was found between eye abnormality and genotype [22].

In a study which evaluated the visual function in 24 patients with NS, it was found that 83% had abnormal results in tests involving ocular movement, acuity, stereopsis. Visual motor integration skills were reported to be significantly impaired in 33%, and 48% had minor impairment when they were asked to copy a set of increasingly complex geometric shapes [28]. In another study, the same author found that children with NS performed worse on tests of form coherence (39% impaired) relative to motion coherence (11% impaired). The authors suggested that children with NS may have great difficulties with ventral stream processing ("what" pathway used for object recognition) compared with dorsal stream processing ("where" pathway used for spatial processing) [29].

A study in adults with NS showed that up to 95% were affected by visual conditions such as strabismus, refractive errors, amblyopia, or nystagmus. Two thirds of patients developed anterior chamber abnormalities including cataracts. Fundoscopic changes were reported in 20% of patients and included optic head drusen, optic disk hypoplasia, and colobomas [30]. In adults with NS, visual motor integration was found to be equivalent to that of adults in the typical group [31].

HEARING IMPAIRMENT

Hearing loss was reported in 40% of the NS patients [17]. This study reevaluated the same cohort of patients 12 years later, and showed that the majority of patients reported normal hearing. Only four patients had hearing loss due to serous otitis media and had unilateral or asymmetric bilateral conductive deafness. A further three patients had sensorineural deafness. Only two patients had mixed conductive and sensorineural hearing loss. None of the patients had cranial imaging to investigate the underlying pathology. One patient with profound sensorineural deafness had a *PTPN11* mutation (A124G) [22].

Another study reported that approximately 10% of affected individuals have auditory deficits in the low frequency range caused by sensorineural hearing loss, and 25% have deficits in the high frequency range [32]. Inner ear structural abnormalities, including temporal bone abnormalities, were reported in these patients [33,34].

NEUROLOGICAL MANIFESTATIONS

Neurological abnormalities and manifestations are not prominent features of NS and are variably present in patients.

A clinical study on 151 subjects with NS, showed that some patients had manifestations in different areas of the nervous system: 94% had abnormal vision or ocular problems, 76% had feeding difficulties, 50% had hypotonia and hypermobility of joints, 40% had abnormal hearing, 13% had recurrent seizures, 3% had hearing loss, and 3% had peripheral neuropathy and an increased incidence of cognitive issues, learning disabilities, and brain abnormalities [17]. Another study reported that 84% of patients had some type of neurological problem [35].

The patients with NS have specific cranial-facial characteristics including triangular shaped face, low hairline, widely spaced eyes, ptosis, and low set ears, but research suggests that structural brain abnormalities are rare. Most frequently seen defects are type I Arnold-Chiari malformations and hydrocephalus [17]. Arnold-Chiari malformation was reported in 11 NS patients. The true incidence is not known and opinions are divided. Some suggest that the observed association may be coincidental [36–39]. Other reported structural abnormalities included: myelomeningocele (in a patient with recurring tethering of the cord), spina bifida occulta, subarachnoid hemorrhage from aneurysm, syringomyelia, optic nerve glioma, medulloblastoma, benign schwannomas or malignant schwannoma [40], and neuroblastoma [41,42]. Association of neurofibromatosis type 1 with NS was also reported [43,44]. Relative megalencephaly, moderately enlarged subarachnoid spaces, and small posterior

Table 1 Neurological features with specific gene mutations

Gene	Developmental	Neurological features
PTPN11	Cognitive impairments, except for N308D and N308S mutations	–
SOS1	Normal or high intelligence	–
RAF1	–	–
KRAS	Severe intellectual disability	–
NRAS	–	Somatic mutations—choroid plexus papilloma, meningioma
BRAF	–	Somatic Mutations—low-grade astrocytomas
RIT-1	–	–
CBL	Developmental delay	Microcephaly
SHOC2	–	Benign external hydrocephalus, cerebellar tonsillar ectopia, periventricular nodular heterotopia, dysplastic corpus callosum
PPP1CB	Global developmental delay, intellectual disability	Macrocephaly
SOS2	–	–
LZTR1	–	Multiple schwannomas
A2ML1	–	–

fossa were reported in a few children with SHOC2 gene mutation [45]. Yet, there is no data to link specific gene mutation to these brain abnormalities (Table 1).

Cerebrovascular anomalies reported were arteriovenous malformations, aneurysms, hypoplasia of the posterior vessels, and Moyamoya [38,46,47].

Neuromuscular abnormalities manifested as abnormal joint hyperextensibility in 75 of 151 patients (50% of cases). Hypotonia was also a common clinical finding. Serum creatine kinase was measured in a cohort of patients, and the concentrations were in the normal range for age and sex. In the same cohort, three adults and one child presented peripheral neuropathy, with distal weakness and altered sensation, in whom spinal cord compression was ruled out and the investigation did not reveal any cause for the neurological findings [17].

Recurrent seizures were reported in 20 of 151 patients (13%) with NS. Grand mal seizures accounted for 14 cases (9%), temporal lobe epilepsy for four cases (3%), and febrile convulsions for two cases (1%) [17]. In the follow up study, in which some of the patients had dropped out, two subjects developed seizures during the follow-up interval, giving a prevalence of 11/112 (10%) in the follow-up sample. The mean age of onset was 11 years in a range of 3–19 years. *PTPN11* mutations were identified in two subjects with seizures [22].

Electroencephalographic (EEG) findings were reported for 28 patients with Noonan syndrome. Twenty (71.4%) of these patients showed EEG abnormalities. The main finding was a diffuse, slow background. They observed diffuse, slow background with focal changes or normal background with focal changes that did not have specific correlation with neurological findings except for a patient with epilepsy, whose EEGs revealed predominantly focal changes. Recurrent seizures were observed in only one patient who also had cortical dysplasia. On the neurological examination, 82% of these patients had various degrees of other neurological abnormalities including slow motor and mental development, spasticity and, in some cases, hypotonia. Their seizures responded well to antiepileptic medications. The researchers concluded that abnormal EEGs should be considered part of the NS [48].

INTELLECTUAL FUNCTIONING, MEMORY, AND ATTENTION

Several studies have shown that while most patients with NS have normal intelligence, the intellectual abilities of NS children are generally lower compared to typical children, and there is a higher risk for intellectual disability.

In a study by Cesarini et al., the IQ scores of NS patients ranged between 70 and 120 [49]. Within the group with normal intelligence, IQ was determined to be 10 points less compared to unaffected siblings or family members and one standard deviation below that of the general population. Most of these patients attended regular education, but between 10% and 40% required special education. According to the researchers, the heterogeneity of the cognitive abilities can be in part attributed to the individual affected genes or types of mutations [49].

It was shown that individuals with most *PTPN11* gene mutations and those without any known mutations more frequently had cognitive impairments than those with SOS1 mutations. However, the N308D and N308S substitution mutations in *PTPN11* were either associated with a mild or no cognitive delays. Whereas SOS1 positive NS individuals had verbal and nonverbal cognitive skills in the average range or higher. Other factors also contributed to differences in cognitive functioning such as motor dexterity, hearing loss, and parental education. Severity of cardiac condition did not seem to play any a role in cognitive functioning [20].

Heterozygous mutations in the *PPP1CB* gene are associated with Noonan syndrome-like disorder with loose anagen hair. The *PPP1CB* gene is highly expressed in the brain throughout the developmental process. Along with other features of NS these mutations have been reported to include global developmental delay and intellectual disability as well [50].

In another study, the IQ scores of children with NS ranged between 64 and 127, with a median of 102. The authors showed that mild intellectual disability was seen in up to 35% of patients. The authors mentioned that the full-scale IQ may shield the possible presence of specific verbal or praxis disabilities [51]. IQ scores in the intellectual disability range (below 70) were reported in 6%–23% of patients with NS [52,53]. Studies on larger groups of young patients with NS did not find differences in intellectual functioning between boys and girls [20].

No significant difference was found between full-scale IQ in a group of adults with NS and community controls matched for age, gender, and education level [54]. About 75% of children with NS perform well in a regular classroom setting and 25% have learning disabilities [19], with 10%–15% of patients requiring special education [52]. Verbal IQ was found to be slightly lower compared to performance IQ [19,55]. Results from a study which administered tests of verbal, visual, and working memory from a standardized memory battery performed by WRAML-2 showed relative strength on verbal memory tasks when compared with visual memory and working memory tasks [56,57]. As with the FS-IQ, in adults with NS there were no significant deficits in delayed verbal recall or delayed visual recall. This finding suggested that memory problems may not be evident in adulthood. It is also possible that adults could be using compensatory strategies to overcome learning and memory deficits [31].

Patients with NS may have attention deficits and attention deficit hyperactivity disorder (ADHD) that may be linked to their academic difficulties. Attention deficits were reported in children with NS in a study by van der Burgt et al. [58]. Other earlier studies, based on parental reports, showed that children with NS have difficulties with attention and hyperactivity when compared to typical children [18,19,52].

A recent study showed that children with NS had higher rates of ADHD diagnosis (31%) than a group of unaffected siblings. According to this study, their attention skills were correlated with their intellectual performance.

This suggests that lower IQ is a risk factor for attention difficulties or that the symptoms of inattention interfere with their cognitive and learning abilities [53].

There was contradicting information regarding auditory and visual memory from two different studies. According to Pierpont et al., children with NS had weaker performance on auditory and visual working memory, with 34% showing significant impairment [57]. Another study reported that adults with NS did not show significant deficits on auditory working memory or other executive functioning tasks compared to the control group, except for self-reported higher rates of subjective executive functioning problems [31].

PSYCHOLOGICAL AND MENTAL HEALTH PROBLEMS

Attention and executive functioning is a common neuropsychological challenge for children with NS [53]. In a study of 32 children and adolescents with NS and their 16 typical siblings, children with NS had higher rates of ADHD and reduced performance compared with unaffected siblings on attention measures.

Adaptive behavior in children with NS is lower compared to age-matched typical children. Younger children had difficulties with motor skills and daily living skills, whereas older children had difficulties with social and communication skills. Researchers did not find differences in motor and daily living skills between boys and girls affected by NS. By school age and adolescence, NS patients showed that these discrepancies between the domains of adaptive functioning disappeared [21].

Social skills are another area where patients with NS have significant difficulties, especially by showing social immaturity and diminished interactions with other children [59,60]. The parents of children with NS also reported more attention seeking behavior compared to typical children that resulted in higher levels of stress in these parents [60].

Children with NS have poor muscle tone, which affects their athletic abilities and decreases their participation in sports, consequently, reducing their opportunities for socialization [5].

Based on checklists, such as the MCHAT (Modified Checklist for Autism in Toddlers), some studies reported an increased level of autism spectrum disorder (ASD) in 12% of children with NS [61]. When these children were evaluated clinically using DSM criteria, none of them met diagnostic criteria for ASD. In another study, 21% of participants with NS showed elevated ASD symptoms, based on screening measures, compared with 0% in a group of their unaffected siblings [62]. Although 12%–21% of patients with NS were reported as having autistic features, most of them did not meet the full diagnostic criteria for ASD.

Adults with NS reported higher levels of difficulties with interpersonal interactions than unaffected adults [54]. Surveyed adults with NS reported that they experienced teasing or bullying as children because they had short stature or looked different compared to their peers [30,55]. As a result of these past experiences, patients with NS may show difficulties with psychological adjustment, depression, social anxiety, impairments of social skills, and academic problems [63]. No particular syndrome causing behavioral disability or psychopathology was observed in patients with NS, and self-esteem was comparable to age-related peers [19].

Reports from studies by Dr. Noonan showed that depression and anxiety may be frequently associated with NS as self-reported by affected adults. In a study of adults with NS [30], 49% reported being diagnosed and taking medications for anxiety and depression [64], but when they were tested using standardized evaluations, no significant differences in depression and anxiety were found between adults with NS and typical adults [54]. Although there are several case reports of patients with NS having different psychiatric disorders, including alcohol abuse, anorexia nervosa, bipolar disorder, panic disorder, obsessive compulsive disorder, and schizophrenia [30,59,65], there is no clear evidence to show that mental illness is more common in adults with NS.

Regarding quality of life based on self-reported questionnaires, no significant differences were found between adults with NS and the general population [55,66], except that NS patients had lower levels of education, graduation, and partnership and higher rates of mortality [55,66].

EVALUATION OF PATIENTS WITH NOONAN SYNDROME

Once a child has been diagnosed with NS, to establish the extent of neurological involvement and the needs of the individual, the following evaluations are recommended: complete physical and neurologic examination, growth parameter plotting on NS growth charts, ophthalmologic evaluation, hearing evaluation, brain and spine MRI if neurologic symptoms are present, multidisciplinary developmental evaluation, and consultation with a clinical geneticist and/or genetic counselor.

MANAGEMENT OF THE DEVELOPMENTAL AND NEUROLOGICAL MANIFESTATIONS OF NOONAN SYNDROME

Given the potential for developmental delays, once the extent of neurological and developmental involvement has been established in a NS patient, early intervention becomes very important to help patients reach their potential. Some patients may require multidisciplinary evaluation and care. Special services which would help affected children include: physical therapy, occupational therapy, speech therapy, special education, social skills, vocational services, and medical management of neurological problems.

Management guidelines were developed by American and European consortia, and the management is optimized to and presented as age-group specific guidelines that emphasize screening and testing for common health issues. There are three papers published with management guidelines/consensus statements: one developed in Europe at the University of Manchester, UK sponsored by DYSCERNE [67]; and two developed in the United States [5,24].

The guidelines are divided into recommendations for four age groups: Neonatal and Infancy (0–1 year old), Childhood (1–11 years old), Adolescence (11–18 years old), and Adulthood (18+ years old). By combining the recommendations from the three papers mentioned earlier, presented here are only those which apply to developmental, neurological, vision, and hearing problems.

I. **Recommendations for the Management of Noonan Syndrome in Neonates and Infancy (0–1 year old)**

In this group, screening is recommended in four areas:

Neuropsychological and behavioral issues: Infants need to be referred for formal developmental assessment during the second half of their first year. If they have delay caused by hypotonia, the patient is recommended management as per the general population. Hypotonia will improve with occupational and physical therapy.

Neurological involvement: Potential complications in infancy include seizures, craniosynostosis, hydrocephalus, and Arnold-Chiari malformation. A low threshold should be considered for investigation of suggestive neurological symptoms (abnormal eye movements, headache, and changes in head circumference) and for referral for brain/spine MRI, if needed.

Vision screening: Anterior or posterior segment ocular abnormalities have been described in NS. Once the diagnosis has been established, infants will need a referral to ophthalmology for baseline evaluation and follow up as deemed appropriate by the ophthalmologist.

Hearing assessment: Infants will need a referral for baseline evaluation during the second half of their first year. Hearing problems should be managed as per the general population.

II. **Recommendations for the Management of Noonan Syndrome in Childhood (1–11 years old)**

Neuropsychological and behavioral issues: Hypotonia and motor delay are common in NS but not necessarily followed by difficulties in adult life. Typically, these will improve with occupational and physical therapy. If the patient has hypermobility, he or she should be referred for occupational therapy.

Screening for developmental delay and speech delay and a full neuropsychological assessment should be done at entry into primary and secondary school, and if/when symptomatic. Management will be as per the general population.

Patients will need an assessment of cognitive abilities, executive function, and attention and learning difficulties. Some patients will need special education and ongoing support for learning and development.

Neurological management: As in the previous age group, a low threshold should be considered for investigation of neurological symptoms that are suggestive of seizures, hydrocephalus, and Arnold-Chiari malformation and for referral for brain/spine MRI, if needed.

Vision screening: Management is the same as for the previous age group. If any vision abnormality is suspected referral recommended, if not already under the care of an ophthalmologist.

Hearing assessment: Patients with NS have an increased risk for conductive hearing loss, but sensorineural hearing loss is rare. Hearing ability needs to be followed on a yearly basis in this age group to prevent speech problems.

III. **Recommendations for the Management of Noonan Syndrome in Childhood (11–18 years old)**

Neuropsychological and behavioral issues: If they have difficulties with daily living or social skills, patients in this age group will benefit from social skills training and programs that teach daily living skills.

Adolescents with NS may develop mood and anxiety disorders and may benefit from psychotherapy or pharmacological management.

Neurology: Individuals are at risk for the same neurological complications: seizures, craniosynostosis, hydrocephalus, and Arnold-Chiari malformation. There are no recommendations for routine screening. If symptomatic, individuals will need to be referred for brain/spine MRI and for management of epilepsy as per the standards for the general population.

Vision screening: Recommendations remain the same as for the other age groups. If individuals with NS are not already under ophthalmologic management, they should be referred to an ophthalmologist, if needed.

IV. **Recommendations for the Management of Noonan Syndrome in Adulthood (18 + years old)**

Neuropsychological and behavioral issues: In adults with NS, neuropsychological assessments may be needed if mood/anxiety problems or if intellectual impairment is suspected. Adult patients need attention and intervention for social skills, as this group is predisposed to social isolation as these patients are at risk of living without a partner. They will need access to support for employment, self-help, and independent living.

Neurology: Possible neurological conditions in adults with NS are the same as those for younger age groups. They will need referral for brain/spine MRI if suspicions for these problems arise. Management will be as per the general population.

Vision screening: Adults with NS can have the same eye and vision problems as at younger ages. If not yet under care, they should be referred to an ophthalmologist for evaluation, if needed.

ACKNOWLEDGMENT

I would like to thank and acknowledge Dr. Anne Tournay, M.D. Professor of Pediatrics, UC Irvine and Pediatric Neurology, Children's Hospital Orange County for critical constructive review of the chapter and for providing valuable input.

REFERENCES

[1] Tartaglia M, Gelb BD, Zenker M. Noonan syndrome and clinically related disorders. Best Pract Res Clin Endocrinol Metab 2011;25(1):161–79. https://doi.org/10.1016/j.beem.2010.09.002.

[2] Mendez HM, Opitz JM. Noonan syndrome: a review. Am J Med Genet 1985;21(3): 493–506. https://doi.org/10.1002/ajmg.1320210312.

[3] Mitin N, Rossman KL, Der CJ. Signaling interplay in Ras superfamily function. Curr Biol 2005;15(14):R563–74. https://doi.org/10.1016/j.cub.2005.07.010.

[4] Schubbert S, Shannon K, Bollag G. Hyperactive Ras in developmental disorders and cancer. Nat Rev Cancer 2007;7(4):295–308. https://doi.org/10.1038/nrc2109.

[5] Roberts AE, Allanson JE, Tartaglia M, Gelb BD. Noonan syndrome. Lancet 2013;381 (9863):333–42. https://doi.org/10.1016/S0140-6736(12)61023-X. [Epub 2013 Jan 10].

[6] Noonan JA, Ehmke DA. Associated non cardiac malformations in children with congenital heart disease. J Pediatr 1963;63:468–70.

[7] Samuels IS, Saitta SC, Landreth GE. MAP'ing CNS development and cognition: an ERKsome process. Neuron 2009;61(2):160–7.

[8] Rubinfeld H, Seger R. The ERK cascade: a prototype of MAPK signaling. Mol Biotechnol 2005;31(2):151–74. https://doi.org/10.1385/MB:31:2:151.

[9] Davis S, Laroche S. Mitogen-activated protein kinase/extracellular regulated kinase signalling and memory stabilization: a review. Genes Brain Behav 2006;5(Suppl. 2):61–72. https://doi.org/10.1111/j.601-183X.2006.00230.x.

[10] Fasano S, Brambilla R. Ras-ERK signaling in behavior: old questions and new perspectives. Front Behav Neurosci 2011;5(79). https://doi.org/10.3389/fnbeh.2011.00079. [eCollection 2011].

[11] Frye RE. RASopathies: a window into the molecular mechanisms underlying neurodevelopmental disorders. Dev Med Child Neurol 2015;57(4):315–6.

[12] Nisbet DL, Griffin DR, Chitty LS. Prenatal features of Noonan syndrome. Prenat Diagn 1999;19(7):642–7.

[13] Houweling AC, de Mooij YM, van der Burgt I, Yntema HG, Lachmeijer AM, Go AT. Prenatal detection of Noonan syndrome by mutation analysis of the PTPN11 and the KRAS genes. Prenat Diagn 2010;30(3):284–6.

[14] Myers A, Bernstein JA, Brennan ML, Curry C, Esplin ED, Fisher J, et al. Perinatal features of the RASopathies: Noonan syndrome, cardiofaciocutaneous syndrome and Costello syndrome. Am J Med Genet A 2014;164A(11):2814–21.

[15] Allanson JE. Noonan syndrome. J Med Genet 1987;24(1):9–13.

[16] Otten BJ, Noordam C. Growth in Noonan syndrome. Horm Res 2009;72(Suppl. 2):31–5.

[17] Sharland M, Burch M, McKenna WM, Paton MA. A clinical study of Noonan syndrome. Arch Dis Child 1992;67(2):178–83.

[18] Wood A, Massarano A, Super M, Harrington R. Behavioural aspects and psychiatric findings in Noonan's syndrome. Arch Dis Child 1995;72(2):153–5.

[19] Lee DA, Portnoy S, Hill P, Gillberg C, Patton MA. Psychological profile of children with Noonan syndrome. Dev Med Child Neurol 2005;47(1):35–8.

[20] Pierpont EI, Pierpont ME, Mendelsohn NJ, Roberts AE, Tworog-Dube E, Seidenberg MS. Genotype differences in cognitive functioning in Noonan syndrome. Genes Brain Behav 2009;8(3):275–82.

[21] Pierpont EI, Ellis Weismer S, Roberts AE, Tworog-Dube E, Pierpont ME, Mendelsohn NJ, et al. The language phenotype of children and adolescents with Noonan syndrome. J Speech Lang Hear Res 2010;53(4):917–32.

[22] Shaw AC, Kalidas K, Crosby AH, Jeffery S, Patton MA. The natural history of Noonan syndrome: a long-term follow-up study. Arch Dis Child 2007;92(2):128–32. https://doi.org/10.1136/adc.2006.104547. [Epub 2006 Sep 21].

[23] Shah N, Rodriguez M, Louis DS, Lindley K, Milla PJ. Feeding difficulties and foregut dysmotility in Noonan's syndrome. Arch Dis Child 1999;81(1):28–31.

[24] Romano AA, Allanson JE, Dahlgren J, Gelb BD, Hall B, Pierpont ME, et al. Noonan syndrome: clinical features, diagnosis, and management guidelines. Pediatrics 2010; 126(4):746–59.

[25] Pierpont EI, Pierpont ME, Mendelsohn NJ, Roberts AE, Tworog-Dube E, Rauen KA, et al. Effects of germline mutations in the Ras/MAPK signaling pathway on adaptive behavior: cardiofaciocutaneous syndrome and Noonan syndrome. Am J Med Genet A 2010;152A(3):591–600.

[26] Selas M, Helland WA. Pragmatic language impairment in children with Noonan syndrome. Clin Linguist Phon 2016;27:1–12.

[27] Marin Lda R, da Silva FT, de Sa LC, Brasil AS, Pereira A, Furquim IM, et al. Ocular manifestations of Noonan syndrome. Ophthalmic Genet 2012;33(1):1–5.

[28] Alfieri P, Cesarini L, Zampino G, Pantaleoni F, Selicorni A, Salerni A, et al. Visual function in Noonan and LEOPARD syndrome. Neuropediatrics 2008;39(6):335–40.

[29] Alfieri P, Cesarini L, De Rose P, Ricci D, Selicorni A, Menghini D, et al. Visual processing in Noonan syndrome: dorsal and ventral stream sensitivity. Am J Med Genet A 2011;155A(10):2459–64.

[30] Noonan JA. Noonan syndrome. In: Goldstein SR, Reynolds CR, editors. Handbook of neurodevelopmental and genetic disorders in adults. New York: The Guilford Press; 2005. p. 308–19.

[31] Wingbermuhle E, Roelofs RL, van der Burgt I, Souren PM, Verhoeven WM, Kessels RP, et al. Cognitive functioning of adults with Noonan syndrome: a case-control study. Genes Brain Behav 2012;11(7):785–93.

[32] Qiu WW, Yin SS, Stucker FJ. Audiologic manifestations of Noonan syndrome. Otolaryngol Head Neck Surg 1998;118(3 Pt 1):319–23.

[33] Cremers CW, van der Burgt CJ. Hearing loss in Noonan syndrome. Int J Pediatr Otorhinolaryngol 1992;23(1):81–4.

[34] Naficy S, Shepard NT, Telian SA. Multiple temporal bone anomalies associated with Noonan syndrome. Otolaryngol Head Neck Surg 1997;116(2):265–7.

[35] Duenas DA, Preissig S, Summitt RL, Wilroy RS, Lemmi H, Dews JE. Neurologic manifestations of the Noonan syndrome. South Med J 1973;66(2):193–6.

[36] Holder-Espinasse M, Winter RM. Type 1 Arnold-Chiari malformation and Noonan syndrome. A new diagnostic feature? Clin Dysmorphol 2003;12(4):275.

[37] Ejarque I, Millan-Salvador JM, Oltra S, Pesudo-Martinez JV, Beneyto M, Perez-Aytes A. Arnold-Chiari malformation in Noonan syndrome and other syndromes of the RAS/MAPK pathway. Rev Neurol 2015;60(9):408–12.

[38] Zarate YA, Lichty AW, Champion KJ, Clarkson LK, Holden KR, Matheus MG. Unique cerebrovascular anomalies in Noonan syndrome with RAF1 mutation. J Child Neurol 2014;29(8):NP13–7.

[39] Keh YS, Abernethy L, Pettorini B. Association between Noonan syndrome and Chiari I malformation: a case-based update. Childs Nerv Syst 2013;29(5):749–52.

[40] Kaplan MS, Opitz JM, Gosset FR. Noonan's syndrome. A case with elevated serum alkaline phosphatase levels and malignant schwannoma of the left forearm. Am J Dis Child 1968;116(4):359–66.

[41] Lopez-Miranda B, Westra SJ, Yazdani S, Boechat MI. Noonan syndrome associated with neuroblastoma: a case report. Pediatr Radiol 1997;27(4):324–6.

[42] Cotton JL, Williams RG. Noonan syndrome and neuroblastoma. Arch Pediatr Adolesc Med 1995;149(11):1280–1.

[43] Buehning L, Curry CJ. Neurofibromatosis-Noonan syndrome. Pediatr Dermatol 1995;12(3):267–71.

[44] Huffmeier U, Zenker M, Hoyer J, Fahsold R, Rauch A. A variable combination of features of Noonan syndrome and neurofibromatosis type I are caused by mutations in the NF1 gene. Am J Med Genet A 2006;140(24):2749–56.

[45] Gripp KW, Zand DJ, Demmer L, Anderson CE, Dobyns WB, Zackai EH, et al. Expanding the SHOC2 mutation associated phenotype of Noonan syndrome with loose anagen hair: structural brain anomalies and myelofibrosis. Am J Med Genet A 2013;161A(10):2420–30.

[46] Schon F, Bowler J, Baraitser M. Cerebral arteriovenous malformation in Noonan's syndrome. Postgrad Med J 1992;68(795):37–40.

[47] Ganesan V, Kirkham FJ. Noonan syndrome and moyamoya. Pediatr Neurol 1997; 16(3):256–8.

[48] Lemmi H, Summitt RL, Wilroy Jr RS, Duenas D. Electroencephalographic Findings in the Noonan Syndrome. Clin Electroencephalogr 1973;4(1):4–8.

[49] Cesarini L, Alfieri P, Pantaleoni F, Vasta I, Cerutti M, Petrangeli V, et al. Cognitive profile of disorders associated with dysregulation of the RAS/MAPK signaling cascade. Am J Med Genet A 2009;149A(2):140–6.

[50] Ma L, Bayram Y, McLaughlin HM, Cho MT, Krokosky A, Turner CE, et al. De novo missense variants in PPP1CB are associated with intellectual disability and congenital heart disease. Hum Genet 2016;135(12):1399–409.

[51] Money J, Kalus Jr ME. Noonan's syndrome. IQ and specific disabilities. Am J Dis Child 1979;133(8):846–50.

[52] van der Burgt I, Thoonen G, Roosenboom N, Assman-Hulsmans C, Gabreels F, Otten B, et al. Patterns of cognitive functioning in school-aged children with Noonan syndrome associated with variability in phenotypic expression. J Pediatr 1999;135(6): 707–13.

[53] Pierpont EI, Tworog-Dube E, Roberts AE. Attention skills and executive functioning in children with Noonan syndrome and their unaffected siblings. Dev Med Child Neurol 2015;57(4):385–92.

[54] Wingbermuhle E, Egger JI, Verhoeven WM, van der Burgt I, Kessels RP. Affective functioning and social cognition in Noonan syndrome. Psychol Med 2012;42(2): 419–26.

[55] Verhoeven W, Wingbermuhle E, Egger J, Van der Burgt I, Tuinier S. Noonan syndrome: psychological and psychiatric aspects. Am J Med Genet A 2008;146A(2):191–6.

[56] Sheslow D, Adams W. Wide range assessment of memory and learning. 2nd ed. Lutz, FL: Psychological Assessment Resources, Inc.

[57] Pierpont EI, Tworog-Dube E, Roberts AE. Learning and memory in children with Noonan syndrome. Am J Med Genet A 2013;161A(9):2250–7.

[58] van der Burgt I. Noonan syndrome. Orphanet J Rare Dis 2007;2:4.

[59] Wingbermuehle E, Egger J, van der Burgt I, Verhoeven W. Neuropsychological and behavioral aspects of Noonan syndrome. Horm Res 2009;72(Suppl. 2):15–23.

[60] Sarimski K. Developmental and behavioural phenotype in Noonan syndrome? Genet Couns 2000;11(4):383–90.

[61] Alfieri P, Piccini G, Caciolo C, Perrino F, Gambardella ML, Mallardi M, et al. Behavioral profile in RASopathies. Am J Med Genet A 2014;164A(4):934–42.

[62] Adviento B, Corbin IL, Widjaja F, Desachy G, Enrique N, Rosser T, et al. Autism traits in the RASopathies. J Med Genet 2014;51(1):10–20.

[63] Pierpont EI. Neuropsychological functioning in individuals with Noonan syndrome: a systematic literature review with educational and treatment recommendations. J Pediatr Neuropsychol 2016;2(1–2):14–33.

[64] Smpokou P, Tworog-Dube E, Kucherlapati RS, Roberts AE. Medical complications, clinical findings, and educational outcomes in adults with Noonan syndrome. Am J Med Genet A 2012;158A(12):3106–11. https://doi.org/10.1002/ajmg.a.35639. [Epub 2012 Nov 19].

[65] Arvaniti A, Samakouri M, Keskeridou F, Veletza S. Concurrence of anorexia nervosa and Noonan syndrome. Eur Eat Disord Rev 2014;22(1):83–5.

[66] Binder G, Grathwol S, von Loeper K, Blumenstock G, Kaulitz R, Freiberg C, et al. Health and quality of life in adults with Noonan syndrome. J Pediatr 2012;161 (3):501–505.e1.

[67] Group D-NSGD. Management of Noonan syndrome: a clinical guideline; 2010.

CHAPTER 8

Hematology/Oncology in Noonan Syndrome

Moran Gotesman*, Amit Soni[†,‡]

*Clinical Assistant Professor of Pediatrics, David Geffen School of Medicine at UCLA Pediatric Hematology/Oncology, Harbor-UCLA Medical Center, Torrance, CA, United States
[†]CHOC Children's Clinic, Orange, CA, United States
[‡]University of California-Irvine, Irvine, CA, United States

Abstract

Since the first hematological abnormalities in Noonan syndrome were first described in 1980, we provide a brief contemporary review of the hematologic and oncologic associations unique to patients with Noonan syndrome. This review highlights the more common associations you are likely to encounter in caring for patients with Noonan syndrome.

Keywords: Hematology abnormalities, Noonan syndrome, Oncology abnormalities, Coagulation, Cancer, Factor XI deficiency, Thrombocytopenia, Platelet dysfunction, PTPN11, RAS, JMML, CBL, Malignancy

Abbreviations

ALL	acute lymphoblastic leukemia
aPTT	activated prothromboplastin time
DNET	dysembryoplastic neuroepithelial tumors
GCL	giant cell lesions
JMML	juvenile myelomonocytic leukemia
MAPK	mitogen-activated protein kinase
NS	Noonan syndrome
PT	prothrombin time
VWD	Von Willebrand disease

COAGULATION ABNORMALITIES

Introduction

The hematological abnormalities in Noonan syndrome (NS) were first described in 1980 by Festen [1] when he described four young boys with Noonan syndrome who underwent orchiectomy procedures and had significant bleeding. However, since then, the relationship between bleeding diatheses and Noonan syndrome has been more clearly elucidated. This clinically important relationship needs to be considered as patients with NS typically undergo numerous surgical interventions. A heterogeneous group of coagulation abnormalities have been described, yet a contribution to overall bleeding is still less clear.

Prevalence

The prevalence of bleeding in patients with Noonan syndrome ranges widely among published data from 20% to 89%. The broad discrepancy lies in the exact definition used to note a bleeding disorder. There are reported patients with a positive bleeding history but with normal coagulation studies as well as those with a negative bleeding history but with abnormal coagulation testing. Briggs and Dickerman [2] reviewed six studies and found that the prevalence of patients with either a bleeding history or abnormal hemostatic labs ranged from 50% to 89%. More specifically, they noted those that had a bleeding history combined with abnormal hemostatic labs comprised 10%–42% of cases. However, each of these studies also reported patients who had bleeding complications with either normal hemostatic labs or no prior bleeding history, emphasizing the importance of obtaining a thorough bleeding history and analyzing the hemostatic labs.

Clinical History

Patients with Noonan syndrome can present with numerous types of bleeding complications. As multiple parts of the hemostatic cascade can be affected, patients with NS can present with platelet dysfunction bleeding (epistaxis, menorrhagia, gingival bleeding, easy bruising, etc.), factor deficiency bleeding (bleeding into joint spaces, retroperitoneum, intramuscular, etc.), or a combination of bleeding complications. In addition, they can present postoperatively with bleeding complications if a bleeding diathesis was not identified prior to the procedure.

Platelets

Thrombocytopenia was the first described hemostatic lab abnormality in patients with Noonan syndrome. Although there have been multiple case series describing this association, this phenomena is not as common as some of the other hemostatic abnormalities. Platelet function analysis has only been reviewed in some case reports. The same review by Briggs and Dickerman analyzed the few studies that assessed platelet dysfunction and reported a prevalence of 27% (16/59). However, a more recent case control study involving 39 patients with NS reported platelet dysfunction in 82.9% of the patients [3].

Von Willebrand Disease

Presumptive Von Willebrand Disease (VWD) was first reported in 1988 by Witt [4] in three patients with Noonan syndrome. Since then only a handful of case series assessed VWF:Ag, VWF:Cof and Factor VIII to be able to make the diagnosis of VWD. Due to lack of data it is difficult to comment on the association of NS with VWD.

Factor Deficiencies

Clotting factor deficiencies are a well-established entity in patients with Noonan syndrome. Factor XI deficiency is the most common and first documented clotting factor deficiency. Reviewing multiple NS cohorts found that Factor XI deficiency is found in approximately 37% of studied patients. (W, S, M, B) Factors XII and VIII are the next most common and are often seen in concordance with Factor XI deficiency. The least common but still identified deficiencies are of Factors V and IX, which are seen commonly in conjunction with the previously described deficiencies.

Recommended Screening Tests

Initial screening coagulation studies should include a prothrombin time (PT), activated prothromboplastin time (aPTT), and a Factor XI activity level. If above PT or PTT times are abnormal, further factor assessment should be undertaken with activities for Factors V, VII, VIII, IX, XII obtained. As deficiency or abnormality of Von Willebrand Factor has not yet been clearly elucidated, a comprehensive vWF panel should be screened as well during initial assessment. Due to the frequency of platelet abnormalities a screening total blood count to assess platelet number and a screening platelet function assay should be done, if parameters are met for accurate results.

Management

The management of patients with Noonan syndrome can be quite complicated considering the multiple bleeding diatheses these patients can present with. For patients who present with bleeding due to unclear etiology, testing should be undertaken to elucidate underlying cause of the bleeding. As factor deficiencies are most prevalent in this population, fresh frozen plasma can be the initial treatment of choice for patients with uncontrolled bleeding.

Cryoprecipate products contain higher concentrations of Factor VIII and vWF. Platelet transfusion should also be considered even if platelet counts are normal due to high rates of platelet dysfunction. The most important step of management is prevention with proper work up prior to procedures or when a diagnosis of NS is made.

CANCER RISK

Introduction

Germline mutations in the RAS-MAPK (mitogen-activated protein kinase) pathway are responsible for Noonan syndrome and other related disorders [5]. Some of these specific genetic mutations are also cancer predisposition genes, thus making patients with NS more susceptible to certain malignancies. The RAS signaling pathway is a major contributor to carcinogenesis. Somatic mutations in *PTPN11*, *KRAS*, *NRAS*, *BRAF*, and *CBL* occur in a broad range of malignancies [6–8]. Both the somatic mutations in the genes involved in the RAS pathway are associated with neoplasms as well as the various developmental syndromes associated with RASopathies or germline mutations carry increased childhood cancer risk. In NS there is a high risk of myeloproliferative disease resembling juvenile myelomonocytic leukemia (JMML), and in other RASopathies, such as Costello syndrome, are predisposed to develop specific malignancies such as embryonal rhabdomyosarcoma, neuroblastoma, and bladder cancer. The first study to quantify the risk of childhood cancer with RASopathies was conducted a large group of investigators in Germany. The authors accessed German Childhood Cancer Registry and analyzed the occurrence of childhood cancer in mutation positive NS as well as other RASopathies. The childhood cancer risk was approximately eightfold in NS [9]. These various cancers include varied categories such as dysembryoplastic neuroepithelial tumors, acute lymphoblastic leukemia, neuroblastoma, and rhabdomyosarcoma (Fig. 1).

Surveillance

In NS patients with specific *PTPN11* or *KRAS* mutations known to be associated with high risk of myeloproliferative therapy/JMML. The recommendations for Cancer Surveillance in Individuals with RASopathies recommend assessing the splenic size along with CBC with differential every 3–6 monthly starting at birth or from the time of diagnosis until age 5 years [10].

No surveillance was recommended for low cancer risk if the childhood cancer risk for less than 5% or unknown but had a low likelihood of

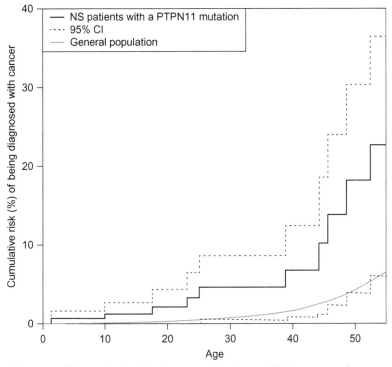

Fig. 1 Age-specific cumulative risk of cancer in patients with Noonan syndrome and a mutation in *PTPN11*. We found a cumulative risk of 23% (95% CI, 7.6%–38.4%) up to age of 55 years, which represents a 3.5-fold increased risk (95% CI, 2.0–5.9) compared with the general population. *(Permission obtained from Jongmans MC, van der Burgt I, Hoogerbrugge PM, Noordam K, Yntema HG, Nillesen WM, et al. Cancer risk in patients with Noonan syndrome carrying a PTPN11 mutation. Eur J Hum Genet 2011;19(8):870–4.)*

occurrence. The guidelines suggested not to do any routine surveillance but should have an increased awareness and low threshold for investigating new potential tumor-related symptoms. These low risk conditions include NS with nonhigh-risk mutations, dysembryoplastic neuroepithelial tumors (DNET), acute lymphoblastic leukemia (ALL), neuroblastoma, and rhabdomyosarcoma [10].

Myeloproliferative Disorder/Juvenile Myelomonocytic Leukemia (JMML)/Acute Lymphoblastic Leukemia (ALL)

Juvenile myelomonocytic leukemia is a rare but aggressive myelodysplastic and myeloproliferative neoplasm of early childhood. It is associated with excessive monocytic and macrophagic proliferation. Patients typically present with splenomegaly, monocytosis, anemia, thrombocytopenia, and elevated fetal hemoglobin [11, 12]. JMML is usually aggressive and necessitates treatment with hematopoietic stem cell transplantation. Patients with Noonan syndrome are at higher risk for the development of JMML, however usually in a form less aggressive and transient.

The heterozygous germline-activating missense mutations *PTPN11* is found in 40% of patients with NS and is the most commonly involved gene [13]. A Netherlands study found a 3.5-fold increased risk of all cancers combined in a cohort of 297 individuals with germline *PTPN11* mutations [14]. Most patients with NS and myeloproliferative disease harbor a *PTPN11* mutation [15], and about 35% of sporadic JMML cases display an acquired somatic *PTPN11* mutation [16]. A French study addressed the association between JMML and NS in a large cohort of 641 patients with germline *PTPN11* mutations. Twenty patients developed JMML [11]. Another study found three cases of JMML among 519 patients with a germline *PTPN11* mutation [9]. Although there is a clear association between *PTPN11* associated NS and JMML, the resulting phenotype is still difficult to predict [11].

Another rare cause of Noonan syndrome is mutations in the tumor suppressor gene *CBL,* which predisposes to JMML. However, this results in an even less severe JMML phenotype [17]. These patients can often time be monitored, and the leukemia self-resolves.

More recently, multiple case reports also show an association between *PTPN11* germline mutations and acute lymphoblastic leukemia [9].

Solid and CNS Tumors

A variety of solid tumors have been reported to be associated with Noonan syndrome, particularly harboring the *PTPN11* gene. A large retrospective review reported on five cases of rhabdomyosarcoma, two of which had the *SOS1* gene mutation, and five cases of neuroblastoma, all having the *PTPN11* mutation [18]. A range of different CNS tumors such as dysembryoplastic neuroepithelial tumor (DNET) are also prevalent and usually found in patients with the *PTPN11* mutations [14, 18, 19].

Management

Patients with Noonan syndrome, particularly with germline RAS pathway mutations, are associated with increased cancer risk than those expected in the general population. However, they are meaningfully lower than those seen in the more familiar adult-onset cancer susceptibility disorders, such as hereditary breast/ovarian cancer and hereditary colorectal cancer [9]. Thus, it appears that germline RAS pathway mutations represent intermediate cancer risk variants, leading to significantly but moderately increased cancer risk.

Due to the heterogeneity and different timing of malignancy presentations, it is difficult to develop a straightforward surveillance program for these patients [14]. The cohort reported by Jongmans et al. showed that there is a 3.5-fold increase in the overall cancer risk up to the age of 55 years in *PTPN11* mutation NS patients.

There have been a cases of tumor growth while they were receiving growth hormone therapy [20]. It is unknown if there is an increase on risk of tumorigenesis or augmentation in the size of the tumors after growth hormone therapy.

Giant Cell Lesions (GCL)

GCL are benign tumor-like lesions most frequently affecting the mandible but also occurring in maxilla and other bones or soft tissues. Histologically these lesions consist of multinucleated giant cells in interspersed with connective fibrous tissue with spindle-shaped mononucleated cells. The process of GCL development can start at a very young age around the third or fourth year of life and progresses until the late adolescents into young adulthood up to 30 years of age. It is more predominant in females and twice more common in the mandibular region than the maxilla [21, 22]. Multiple or multifocal GCL are rare and other conditions such as primary hyperparathyroidism needs to be excluded.

The pathogenesis of GCL formation is incompletely understood. The pathophysiological link seems to be the proliferation of tumor cells as mononucleated osteoblast-like cell activity leading to increased cytokine production and maturation of a subset of mononuclear phagocytes into osteoclast-like giant cells.

In the clinical course GCLs can be aggressive or nonaggressive. The nonaggressive form has a slow growing pattern and painless swelling. The aggressive form is associated with rapid growth, pain, paresthesia, tooth root resorption, cortical bone resorption, and high recurrence rates even after surgical treatment.

The GCLs on imaging present as multiloculated in the right mandible with cortical thinning of the buccal and lingual cortex. Radiological features X-ray reveals multilocular cystic changes, expansive lesions. In the mandibular and maxillary bones secondary tooth resorption can also be present or is spared.

The common treatment of GCL is surgery; the techniques include simple curettage, curettage with peripheral osteotomy, en bloc resection (5 mm surgical margins), and cryosurgery. In children, nonsurgical approach should be considered.. The nonsurgical treatments included subcutaneous alpha interferon, intranasal and SQ calcitonin and corticosteroid injections, but no specific therapeutic option has been well described for NS [23].

The clinical picture could be very similar to cherubism which can be caused by mutations in the *SH3BP2* gene. The GCLs in NS are distinct from cherubism and none have SH3BP2 gene mutations. *PTPN11* mutations have been reported in giant cell lesions (GCL) in NS [24]. But in NS certain mutations in *PTPN11* gene has been found to be associated with GCL; another genetic etiology of the NS is *SOS1* gene mutations, which is also associated with GCLs [25]. The giant cell lesions are likely to be a part of the spectrum cases of Noonan syndrome. It is hypothesized that the multiple giant cell lesions suggest the second hit in the genes involved in RAS MAPK pathway. Although the genetic mechanism of giant cell lesion development is unclear.

Growth hormone is frequently used in Noonan syndrome for treatment of short stature. In those specific high risk *PTPN11* or *KRAS* gene mutations which increases the predisposition or high risk for the development of malignancies and decision should be done an individual basis and appropriate surveillance and monitoring needs to be undertaken [26].

REFERENCES

[1] Festen C. An unusual complication of orchidopexia in Noonan's syndrome. Chir Pediatr 1980;2(6):393–5.
[2] Briggs BJ, Dickerman JD. Bleeding disorders in Noonan syndrome. Pediatr Blood Cancer 2012;58:167–72.
[3] Artoni A, Selicorni A, Passamonti SM, Lecchi A, Bucciarelli P, Cerutti M, Cianci P, Gianniello F, Martinelli I. Hemostatic abnormalities in Noonan syndrome. Pediatrics 2014;133:e1299–304.
[4] Witt DR, McGillvray BC, Allanson JE, et al. Bleeding diathesis in Noonan syndrome: a common association. Am J Med Genet 1988;31:305–17.
[5] Lepri FR, Scavelli R, Digilio MC, et al. Diagnosis of Noonan syndrome and related disorders using target next generation sequencing. BMC Med Genet 2014;15:14.
[6] Downward J. Signal transduction. Prelude to an anniversary for the RAS oncogene. Science 2006;314(5798):433–4.
[7] Makishima H, Cazzolli H, Szpurka H, et al. Mutations of e3 ubiquitin ligase cbl family members constitute a novel common pathogenic lesion in myeloid malignancies. J Clin Oncol 2009;27(36):6109–16.

[8] Schubbert S, Shannon K, Bollag G. Hyperactive Ras in developmental disorders and cancer. Nat Rev Cancer 2007;7(4):295–308.

[9] Kratz CP, Franke L, Peters H. Cancer spectrum and frequency among children with Noonan, Costello, and cardio-facio-cutaneous syndromes. Br J Cancer 2015;112: 1392–7. https://doi.org/10.1038/bjc.2015.75.

[10] Villani A, Greer MC, Kalish JM, Nakagawara A, Nathanson KL, Pajtler KW, et al. Recommendations for cancer surveillance in individuals with RASopathies and other rare genetic conditions with increased cancer risk. Clin Cancer Res 2017;23(12):e83–90.

[11] Strullu M, Caye A, Lachenaud J, et al. Juvenile myelomonocytic leukaemia and Noonan syndrome. J Med Genet 2014;51(10):689–97.

[12] Loh ML. Recent advances in the pathogenesis and treatment of juvenile myelomonocytic leukaemia. Br J Haematol 2011;152:677–87.

[13] Romano AA, Allanson JE, Dahlgren J, et al. Noonan syndrome: clinical features, diagnosis, and management guidelines. Pediatrics 2010;126:746–59.

[14] Jongmans MC, van der Burgt I, Hoogerbrugge PM, Noordam K, Yntema HG, Nillesen WM, Kuiper RP, Ligtenberg MJ, van Kessel AG, van Krieken JH, Kiemeney LA, Hoogerbrugge N. Cancer risk in patients with Noonan syndrome carrying a PTPN11 mutation. Eur J Hum Genet 2011;19(8):870–4.

[15] Kratz CP, Niemeyer CM, Castleberry RP, Cetin M, et al. The mutational spectrum of PTPN11 in juvenile myelomonocytic leukemia and Noonan syndrome/myeloproliferative disease. Blood 2005;106:2183–5.

[16] Pérez B, Kosmider O, Cassinat B, et al. Genetic typing of CBL, ASXL1, RUNX1, TET2 and JAK2 in juvenile myelomonocytic leukaemia reveals a genetic profile distinct from chronic myelomonocytic leukaemia. Br J Haematol 2010;151:460–8.

[17] Niemeyer CM, Kang MW, Shin DH, Loh ML. Germline CBL mutations cause developmental abnormalities and predispose to juvenile myelomonocytic leukemia. Nat Genet 2010;42(9):794–800.

[18] Smpokou P, Zan DJ, Rosenbaum KN, Summar ML. Malignancy in Noonan syndrome and related disorders. Clin Genet 2015;88:516–22.

[19] Selter M, Dresel R, Althaus J, Baz Bartels M, Dittrich S, Geb S, Hoche F, Qirshi M, Vlaho S, Zielen S, Kieslich M. Dysembryoplastic neuroepithelial tumor (DNET) in a patient with Noonan syndrome. Neuropediatrics 2010;41:P1356.

[20] McWilliams GD, SantaCruz K, Hart B, Clericuzio C. Occurrence of DNET and other brain tumors in Noonan syndrome warrants caution with growth hormone therapy. Am J Med Genet A 2016;170(1):195–201.

[21] Bernaerts A, Vanhoenacker FM, Hintjens J, Chapelle K, Salgado R, De Foer B, et al. Tumors and tumor-like lesions of the jaw: radiolucent lesions. JBR BTR 2006;89(2): 81–90.

[22] Orhan E, Erol S, Deren O, Sevin A, Ekici O, Erdogan B. Idiopathic bilateral central giant cell reparative granuloma of jaws: a case report and literature review. Int J Pediatr Otorhinolaryngol 2010;74(5):547–52.

[23] Bufalino A, Carrera M, Carlos R, Coletta RD. Giant cell lesions in Noonan syndrome: case report and review of the literature. Head Neck Pathol 2010;4(2):174–7.

[24] Tartaglia M, Kalidas K, Shaw A, Song X, Musat DL, van der Burgt I, et al. PTPN11 mutations in Noonan syndrome: molecular spectrum, genotype-phenotype correlation, and phenotypic heterogeneity. Am J Hum Genet 2002;70(6):1555–63.

[25] Hanna N, Parfait B, Talaat IM, Vidaud M, Elsedfy HH. SOS1: a new player in the Noonan-like/multiple giant cell lesion syndrome. Clin Genet 2009;75(6):568–71.

[26] Raman S, Grimberg A, Waguespack SG, Miller BS, Sklar CA, Meacham LR, et al. Risk of neoplasia in pediatric patients receiving growth hormone therapy—a report from the Pediatric Endocrine Society Drug and Therapeutics Committee. J Clin Endocrinol Metab 2015;100(6):2192–203.

FURTHER READING

[27] Collins E, Turner G. The Noonan syndrome—a review of the clinical and genetic features of 27 cases. J Pediatr 1973;83:941–50.

[28] de Haan M, Kamp JJP, Briet E, Dubbeldam J. Noonan syndrome: partial factor XI deficiency. Am J Med Genet 1988;29:277–82.

[29] Sharland M, Patton M, Chittolie A, et al. Coagulation factor abnormalities in Noonan syndrome. J Med Genet 1990;27:646.

[30] Sharland M, Patton MA, Talbot S, et al. Coagulation—factor deficiencies and abnormal bleeding in Noonan's syndrome. Lancet 1992;339:19–21.

[31] Massarano AA, Wood A, Tait RC, et al. Noonan syndrome: coagulation and clinical aspects. Acta Paediatr 1996;85:1181–5.

[32] Bertola DR, Carneiro JDA, D'Amico EA, et al. Hematological findings in Noonan syndrome. Rev Hosp Clin Fac Med Sao Paulo 2003;58:5–8.

[33] Kitchens CS, Alexander JA. Partial deficiency of coagulation factor XI as newly recognized feature of Noonan syndrome. J Pediatr 1983;102:224–7.

[34] Tosetto A, Rodeghiero F, Castaman G, et al. A quantitative analysis of bleeding symptoms in type 1 von Willebrand disease: results from a multicenter European study (MCMDM-1 VWD). J Thromb Haemost 2006;4:766–73.

CHAPTER 9

Analgesia, Anesthesia, and Perioperative Considerations in Noonan Syndrome

Shalini Shah

Department of Anesthesiology & Division of Pain Management, University of California, Irvine, Orange, CA, United States

Abbreviations

ERK	extracellular signal regulated kinases
HCM	hypertrophic obstructive cardiomyopathy
MAPK	mitogen–activated protein kinases
NS	Noonan syndrome
PS	pulmonary stenosis

Abstract

Noonan syndrome (NS) is one of the more common genetic conditions with an estimated prevalence of 1:1000 to 1:2500 births inherited in an autosomal dominant fashion. The main features are the presence of characteristic facial features, cardiac or musculoskeletal abnormalities, and hematological abnormalities which all can impact on perioperative care. The potential anesthetic issues presented by patients with NS relate to impairment of cardiopulmonary function, possibility of a difficult airway, and potential technical difficulty performing regional anesthesia. For example, use of regional and spinal anesthesia would be avoided in the presence of a hypertrophic obstructive cardiomyopathy (HCM) or pulmonary stenosis, respectively. Regional has more chances of complications due to spinal or vertebral anomalies. General anesthesia would be preferred in cases if regional or spinal cannot be performed safely. The problems of anesthesia related to NS need to be determined and assessed preoperatively to avoid complications. Pain disorders are frequent and under-recognized clinical feature of NS. A variety of skeletal abnormalities include congenital spinal deformity, thoracic lordosis, scoliosis, single thoracic curve, single thoracolumbar curve, and double major curve, all of which increases the need for surgical interventions and anesthesia risk.

Keywords: Noonan syndrome, Airway anomalies, Pulmonary stenosis, General anesthesia, Regional anesthesia

INTRODUCTION

Noonan syndrome (NS) is an autosomal dominant condition with an incidence of 1:1000 to 1:2500 live births. Majority of children with NS have congenital heart defects, chest deformities such as pectus excavatum or pectus carinatum, cryptorchidism, hematological disorders, facial dysmorphology, webbed neck, cervical spine anomalies, and kyphoscoliosis which are associated with increased risk of complications from various anesthesia procedures and anesthetic agents. The reported experience of anesthesia use in NS is limited. They are at higher risk for developing hypertensive crisis and urgency. Patients also have to undergo repeated surgical procedures, which further increase the risk of complications. NS is also associated with mild intellectual deficits. Various anesthetic agents such as N-methyl-D-aspartate receptor (NMDAR) antagonists, ketamine, and γ-aminobutyric acid type A receptor (GABAR) agonists have been associated with potential neurotoxic effects on the developing mammalian brain [1]. Patients with NS often require repeated general anesthesia for various surgical procedures [2]. Repeated exposure can potentially lead to apoptosis in brain cells, but it is unknown at this time if repeated exposure to anesthetics can potentially influence the intellectual development. The presence of webbed neck and remnants of lymphedema around the neck presents with potential difficult airway. In the neonatal period, babies with NS can present with a fatal type of lymphangiectasis resulting in persistent pleural effusions [3]. In this chapter, we will review some of the commonly reported anesthetic and perioperative complications in NS of which the anesthesiologists, surgeons, urologists, hematologists, cardiologists, obstetricians, and endocrinologists need to be aware while preparing these patients for surgical procedures.

Increasing number of NS mothers are undergoing pregnancy and parturition. Such situations call for an advanced planning between obstetricians, cardiologist, and anesthesiologists. All risk factors should be discussed with patient, and alternative methods of management should be discussed. Spinal anesthesia should be avoided in conditions with cardiac conditions which are common in NS. Regional anesthesia, although potentially difficult due to vertebral abnormalities, is a safe alternative compared to general anesthesia [4]. But in cases of kyphoscoliosis, lumbar lordosis, relatively narrow spinal canal along with cardiac lesions, general anesthesia has been used and described.

CARDIAC CONSIDERATIONS

The two cardiac lesions most common in NS with anesthetic implications are pulmonary valve stenosis (PS) is present in approximately 80% of patients and hypertrophic obstructive cardiomyopathy (HCM) is present in approximately 30%. PS is also associated with dysplastic pulmonary valves, patent foramen ovale. Therefore, air should be carefully removed from all intravenous lines and syringes. HCM increases the susceptibility of developing acute congestive heart failure because of the hemodynamic fluctuations in the operative period. NS could present a challenge to an experienced cardiac anesthesiologist due to the presence of difficult airway, pulmonary stenosis, webbed neck along with the existence of various other cardiac lesions [5].

Even in the setting HCM, intravenous fluids can be started even a day before surgery and anesthesia can be induced by using higher dosing of Fentanyl and Midazolam and then maintained with Propofol at a rate of 8 mg/kg/h, Fentanyl, Ketamine, and Sevoflurane [6].

The detailed management of the first case of use of general anesthesia in a child with cardiomyopathy was described by Campbell et al. The patient was a 5-year-old female with a history of NS, HCM with impaired cardiopulmonary function and difficult airway. At first, the myelography procedure was started after the infusion of 100 ml of plasma expander and then anesthesia was induced with 50 mg of Thiopentone and 7.5 mg of Atracurium. Patient was manually ventilated with 35% FiO_2 and nitrous oxide, followed by 150 mCg of Alfentanil. The trachea was intubated easily with a 5.0 mm plain oral Flexometallic (Mallinckrodt) tracheal tube. Anesthesia was maintained with 35% FiO_2 and nitrous oxide and isoflurane 0.5%. The lungs were gently inflated by hand using a T-piece system to maintain the end-tidal CO_2 between 4 and 5 kPa. Vitals such as heart rate, blood pressure, and oxygen saturations remained within normal limits during induction of anesthesia and throughout the duration of the procedure. Neuromuscular blockade was reversed using 0.75 mg of Neostigmine and 0.3 mg of Atropine. The patient was extubated without issues, and postoperatively the patient did not experience any complications [7].

During the second procedure of subsequent lumbar laminectomy, the patient was premedicated with 36 mg of Trimeprazine and 3.6 mg of Droperidol. For induction of anesthesia, 30 mCg of Fentanyl was given and then followed by intubation. Anesthesia was maintained with nitrous oxide and halothane. The patient was positioned prone on bolsters. Intraoperative analgesia was provided by Diamorphine infused at a rate of 0.3 mCg/kg/min and this infusion was continued to provide postoperative analgesia. The patient stayed in the PICU for recovery and was discharged home after 10 days [7].

Another case of use of general anesthesia was described in a 42-year-old man with a phenotype of NS and on long-term antidepressants (amitriptyline) use was scheduled for operation for ventral hernia. The patient described was a difficult intubation due to facial and spinal abnormalities. He had a history of previous general anesthetic use and been successfully intubated with fiber optic bronchoscopy. The patient was premedicated with Midazolam 3 mg, Fentanyl 50 mCg, and Droperidol 1.25 mg, and intubated awake under bronchofiberscopy after topical Lidocaine 400 mg. Once endotracheal tube placement was confirmed by Thiopental 125 mg and Sevoflurane 0.4% was administered. The patient developed hypotension after intubation which was treated with Ephedrine. After the start of surgery, the blood pressure increased to normal and remained within normal limits until the end of surgery [8].

A majority of NS patients have pulmonary stenosis which increases the right ventricular failure risk if the patient becomes volume overloaded. Therefore, increasing intravascular volume with crystalloid infusions prior to regional or neuraxial anesthesia should only be done with caution. Hypoxia should be avoided in these patients and monitoring of CVP should be considered [7]. If the patients are dehydrated prior to administration of spinal or epidural, block can result in hypotension from the sympathetic blockage, which leads to decrease in right ventricular output and cardiac arrest. In one of the initial cases of NS, patients have been reported to require more circulatory and ventilatory support [9–11]. NS patients also have a higher risk of developing endocarditis involving the mitral and aortic valves [12]. Therefore, they should be consulted by the cardiologist to satisfy the need for prophylactic antibiotics coverage with either amoxicillin or clindamycin (for penicillin allergy).

Transesophageal echocardiography (TEE) has been used preoperatively for detection of cardiac anomalies and new findings. TEE can also be used intraoperatively for cardiac procedures and monitoring in the postoperative period [13].

AIRWAY MANAGEMENT

As anesthesiologist we are very aware of the use of the Mallampati score or classification, which is used to predict the ease of intubation. It can also be used to predict whether the patient has risk for obstructive sleep apnea. The Mallampati scores in NS are reported to range from II to IV, which implies most NS individuals have difficult airway due to presence of webbed neck as a result of remnants of lymphedema. Tracheal intubation would require an aid of a bougie [14]. Various other methods used to secure the upper airway have been reported in NS due to difficult airway issues. These include intubation with awake direct laryngoscopy can be used atypical facial features [15]. Dental treatment under general anesthesia with nasotracheal intubation under curve-tipped suction catheter guidance or insertion of a reinforced laryngeal mask airway has also been done in NS [2].

PULMONARY RISK

Lymph system abnormalities such as generalized or peripheral lymphedema, pulmonary, and intestinal lymphangiectasia can found in 20% of patients with NS patients [16]. Bronchial cast or plastic bronchitis has been reported in patients with NS undergoing surgical repair for heart defects and it presents as life threatening emergency. Histopathology report of the tissue consists of neutrophils, alveolar macrophages, fibrinous and mucinous material called bronchial cast, leading to obstruction of the large airways, and development of plastic bronchitis [17, 18]. The mechanism of formation of the cast is linked to high pulmonary or intrathoracic lymphatic pressure and/ or presence of undetected lymphobronchial fistulae and the constitution is similar to lymphatic material [19]. Bronchial casts can clinically present as respiratory distress along with and coughing up of "chicken meat" or "noodles" like substance [20]. Bronchial casts usually occur following surgery for congenital cardiac defects resulting in higher mortality rates [17].

HEMATOLOGICAL COMPLICATIONS

NS is also at higher risk of Factor XI deficiency and thrombocytopenia. Clotting and platelet defects considerably restrict the possible analgesic and anesthetic options in patients with NS [15]. These could raise difficulties with development of epidural hematoma after epidural analgesia.

Postsurgical bleeding interventions was reported in 5/33, which is approximately 15.2% of NS patients [21]. In patients undergoing surgery, the rate of bleeding was much higher at the rate of 45% and these include mild–to–moderate bleeding diathesis scores. These patients had documented coagulation or platelet abnormalities. Postsurgical bleeding was only limited to minor diathesis if patients did not have predetermined defects. Hence, preoperative screening of patients with NS for bleeding diathesis is imperative for surgical risk assessment [21]. The use of aspirin and other nonsteroidal antiinflammatory drugs was avoided in these patient with NS and bleeding tendencies [22].

PTPN11 gene mutations which are associated with pulmonary stenosis and are more prone to the shear stress-related destruction of the von Willebrand factor (vWF) as an important hemostatic component, and the deficiency of vWF. Results in prolonged bleeding time and can lead to delayed bleeding or serious postsurgical hemorrhage. In a specific case, Desmopressin was administered preoperatively to increase platelet aggregation and the vWF levels.

In NS preoperative management, guidelines for hematologic screening exist. Each patient should undergo first and second tier of hematological screening. First tier of testing includes a CBC with differential count and prothrombin time (PT)/activated partial thromboplastin time (aPTT). The second tier of testing should be performed in consultation with a hematologist; these include specific factor activity for factor XI, factor XII, factor IX, factor VIII, vWF, and testing of platelet function such as bleeding time or platelet aggregation studies [23]. For details about hematological manifestations, please review Chapter 8.

NS with *PTPN11* gene mutations result in a higher risk of malignancies, particularly hematological malignancies [24]. In particular, malignant mastocytosis can create a major concern for anesthesiologists due to the increased number of histamine-filled mast cells as some anesthetic drugs cause histamine release [22]. Care should be taken to avoid histamine releasing drugs such as Vecuronium, Pancuronium, Mivacurium, and Atracurium in these patients. Each drug was added to or eliminated from the anesthetic plan to prevent histamine release by the activation of triggers.

OBSTETRICS ANESTHESIA

Pregnancy presents additional concerns for Cesarean delivery in a parturient mother with NS. The course during pregnancy can be complicated with pulmonary edema and tachycardia in expectant mother; which has resulted in intrauterine fetal demise [25]. Pregnancy and delivery in NS should be considered a high-risk case from early pregnancy. The anesthesiologist should prepare for a difficult airway, cardio-valvular anomalies, cardiopulmonary abnormalities, spine alignment concerns, and short stature. Assessment of these features is important in the preoperative consultation to better prepare for anesthetic needs during delivery [11, 25, 26]. During pregnancy, the cardiac defect of HCM would worsen especially with interventricular septum hypertrophy leading to left ventricular outflow obstruction with mostly a normal left ventricular systolic function. There are currently only a few number of reported NS cases regarding the choice of anesthesia use in labor and delivery. Most of these reports discuss the use of general anesthesia and the mode of delivery is C-section [4]. There is one reported case of use of epidural labor analgesia in a C-section and the only another use of epidural resulting in a successful vaginal delivery [26]. In such a case of C-section, epidural anesthesia and analgesia were preferred to general anesthesia due to the possibility of difficult intubation as a result of high-arched palate, micrognathia, and short-webbed neck [26].

Short stature and potential skeletal anomalies (pectus excavatum, pectus carinatum, and kyphoscoliosis) in NS increase the risk of cardiopulmonary compromise during pregnancy and delivery. The functional residual capacity (FRC) which is decreased in pregnancy is compromised even further in NS.

In a published case report, a 20-year-old pregnant female with extreme short stature could not undergo normal vaginal delivery as the pelvis was flat and contracted resulting in a cephalopelvic disproportion. As a result, she underwent a C-section. Regional anesthesia was attempted and due to the difficulty of location the epidural space subarachnoid block was performed at L3–4 interspace in right lateral position. Once the needle was secured 10 mg of hyperbaric Tetracaine was given. The patient was placed supine with left uterine displacement. Due to kyphoscoliosis, the level of anesthesia rose from T4 to T2. By the end of C-section, it had raised to level of T1 resulting in hypotension. The blood pressure eventually stabilized with aggressive crystalloid and 10 mg doses of IV Ephedrine [11]. Thus, regional anesthesia should be used with caution in patients with kyphoscoliosis.

MALIGNANT HYPERTHERMIA

There have been few cases of malignant hyperthermia (MH) which developed during the induction of general anesthesia or postoperatively in patients with NS like phenotype [27–30]. Some of these earlier reports of MH could have been in similar phenotypic features of patients with King-Denborough syndrome which is associated with congenital myopathy, skeletal abnormalities and dysmorphic features, and characteristic facial appearance. King-Denborough syndrome is known to be associated with MH. There was one case of MH in the 60 patients included in the cited study by Lee et al. [31]. MH is a serious complication from anesthesia, but it is not certain if all patients with NS should be considered at risk for the development of this complication. In NS individuals with skeletal myopathy, normal to elevated creatine phosphokinase (CPK) levels plus HCM, the avoidance of anesthetics associated with MH should be considered [23]. Preoperative assessment should include to check if skeletal muscle biopsy in individuals with high risk of skeletal or cardiac myopathy has been considered to look for presence of excess muscle spindle in patients with phenotype described earlier.

NOONAN SYNDROME AND PAIN

Pain is a frequent and under-recognized clinical feature of NS. Individuals with NS reported problems related to pain, decreased muscle strength, fatigue, and clumsiness, which had an evident impact on functioning in daily life. In a focus group, interviews with people with NS and their relatives expressed that the healthcare professionals were not receptive toward them when it came to understand their motor performance problems [32]. Most of the motor performance improved with exercise and physiotherapy interventions. A study published the results of the questionnaire about pain among NS individuals. Among these, 53% were females. The mean age was 17 years and approximately half of them had a *PTPN11* gene mutation. A surprising high proportional number of patients close to 62% experienced chronic pain. There was a significant relationship between prevalence of pain and residing in a cold climate ($P = .004$). Most of the chronic pain occurred in extremities, joints, head, and trunk. But the pain was more significantly common in extremities and joints. The individuals with hypermobility were more likely to experience pain [33].

A recently published study confirms that motor performance, strength, and endurance are significantly impaired in children with NS. The authors reported 19 children with an age ranges from 6 years to 11 years were assessed. More than 60% of the parents of the children reported pain, decreased muscle strength, reduced endurance, and/or clumsiness in daily functioning. These children were found to have higher presence of generalized hypermobility along with significantly lower grip strength, muscle force, and 6-min walking test. It was strongly recommended that children with NS should referred to early physical and/or occupational therapy [34].

Orthopedic manifestations occur frequently in RAS/MAPK(ERK) disorders and can be used in phenotypic differentiation between these disorders. In a prospective study, 26 individuals with NS were evaluated by an orthopedic surgeon and clinical geneticist. They have a high instance of serious cervical spine disorders, including cervical stenosis, Arnold–Chiari malformation, and syringomyelia. In this cohort, 81% of patients had history of chronic pain, approximately 42% had pes planus, 19% reported pes cavus, 19% had hip contractures, and 12% had hand dysfunction along with 8% patients had hip dysplasia [35]. A cross-sectional study which reported the prevalence of both orthopedic conditions such as scoliosis and chronic joint pain was 54% each in a cohort of 35 adolescents and adults aged 16–68 years old. The genetic profile of this cohort was as follows with 37% were *PTPN11* positive, 23% were *SOS1* positive, and 3% were *BRAF* positive [36].

SKELETAL ABNORMALITIES

Apart from cardiovascular and airway abnormalities, skeletal abnormalities, especially of the spine have also been described. However, no detailed and systematic study of such spinal deformities has been presented in the literature. Spinal deformities are present is approximately one-third of patients which include congenital spinal deformity, thoracic lordosis, scoliosis, single thoracic curve, single thoracolumbar curve, and double major curve. These deformities present in prepubertal age group and majority of them required surgical correction for scoliosis and associated thoracic lordosis [31]. Scoliosis with an associated thoracic lordosis occurs more frequently in NS and relatively early and severe. Spinal X-ray should be done for early detection and treatment of spinal deformity. Regional anesthesia in NS is challenging due to the higher incidence of kyphoscoliosis and increased curvature of the spine. Accessing the epidural space can impose challenges. In addition, the level of anesthesia would be difficult to control.

SUMMARY

In individuals with confirmed or suspected NS, the use of regional anesthesia should be given a consideration but has to be carried out with caution and an ENT surgeon should be available until the level of anesthesia is attained. Regional anesthesia can avoid the risks associated with difficult intubations and aspiration. However, anesthesiologists should also be aware of the increased incidence of kyphoscoliosis and lumbar lordosis so accessing the epidural space can impose challenges. Spinal anesthesia should be avoided in conditions with cardiac conditions such as pulmonic valve stenosis, which is commonly seen in NS. In parturient NS, both general and regional anesthesia have been undertaken. As discussed, NS has been associated with bleeding diathesis, hence all patients with NS should undergo a preoperative evaluation (first- and second-tier testing) of bleeding risk. The first tier of testing includes a CBC with differential, PT, and aPTT. The second tier involves testing for the specific factor deficiency which has to be performed in consultation with a hematologist. Interventional cardiac catheterization or open-heart surgery carries higher risk due to the bleeding tendencies. Individuals with phenotypic characteristics similar to NS and some individuals with NS could be at higher risk for MH when receiving general anesthesia. Avoidance of anesthetics associated with MH should be considered in certain cases.

ACKNOWLEDGMENT

I would like to thank and acknowledge Dr. Ashley Broussard, M.D. Professor of Anesthesiology, UC Irvine for critical constructive review of the chapter and for providing valuable input.

REFERENCES

[1] Sun L. Early childhood general anaesthesia exposure and neurocognitive development. Br J Anaesth 2010;105:61–8 (Suppl.).
[2] Asahi Y, Fujii R, Usui N, Kagamiuchi H, Omichi S, Kotani J. Repeated general anesthesia in a patient with Noonan syndrome. Anesth Prog 2015;62(2):71–3.
[3] Ford JJ, Trotter CW. Noonan syndrome complicated by primary pulmonary lymphangiectasia. Neonatal Netw 2015;34(2):117–25. https://doi.org/10.1891/0730-832.34.2.117.
[4] Magboul MM. Anaesthetic management of emergency caesarean section in a patient with Noonan's syndrome-case report and literature review. Middle East J Anaesthesiol 2000;15(6):611–7.
[5] Bajwa SJ, Gupta S, Kaur J, Panda A, Bajwa SK, Singh A, et al. Anesthetic considerations and difficult airway management in a case of Noonan syndrome. Saudi J Anaesth 2011;5 (3):345–7.
[6] Nakagawa M, Kinouchi K, Matsunami K, Ono R, Miyagawa Y, Ueda D, et al. Anesthetic management of a child with Noonan syndrome and hypertrophic obstructive cardiomyopathy. Masui 2006;55(1):92–5.
[7] Campbell AM, Bousfield JD. Anaesthesia in a patient with Noonan's syndrome and cardiomyopathy. Anaesthesia 1992;47(2):131–3.
[8] Nakamura S, Takeda K, Nishiyama T, Hanaoka K. General anesthesia for a patient with Noonan's syndrome and long-term antidepressant therapy. Masui 2005;54(8):901–3.
[9] Walts LF, Finerman G, Wyatt GM, Forsythe AB, Moore G. Anaesthesia for dwarfs and other patients of pathological small stature. Can Anaesth Soc J 1975;22(6):703–9.
[10] Cohen SE. Anesthesia for cesarean section in achondroplastic dwarfs. Anesthesiology 1980;52(3):264–6.

[11] Dadabhoy ZP, Winnie AP. Regional anesthesia for cesarean section in a parturient with Noonan's syndrome. Anesthesiology 1988;68(4):636–8.

[12] Chase CJ, Holak EJ, Pagel PS. Anesthetic implications of emergent cesarean section in a parturient with Noonan syndrome and bacterial endocarditis. J Clin Anesth 2013;25 (5):403–6.

[13] Aggarwal V, Malik V, Fau Kapoor PM, PM K, Fau Kiran U, Kiran U. Noonan syndrome: an anesthesiologist's perspective. Ann Card Anaesth 2011;14(3):214–7. https://doi.org/10.4103/0971-9784.84024.

[14] Samra T, Banerjee N. Anaesthesia for emergency ventriculo-peritoneal shunt in an adolescent with Noonan's syndrome. Indian J Anaesth 2014;58(4):452–5.

[15] Grange CS, Heid R, Lucas SB, Ross PL, Douglas MJ. Anaesthesia in a parturient with Noonan's syndrome. Can J Anaesth 1998;45(4):332–6.

[16] Hernandez RJ, Stern AM, Rosenthal A. Pulmonary lymphangiectasis in Noonan syndrome. AJR Am J Roentgenol 1980;134(1):75–80.

[17] Brogan TV, Finn LS, Pyskaty Jr. DJ, Redding GJ, Ricker D, Inglis A, et al. Plastic bronchitis in children: a case series and review of the medical literature. Pediatr Pulmonol 2002;34(6):482–7.

[18] Jagtap SR, Iyer HR, Bakhshi RG, Lahoti HN. Post-operative airway obstruction in Noonan syndrome: an unusual presentation. Indian J Anaesth 2015;59(7):442–4. https://doi.org/10.4103/0019-5049.160961.

[19] Shah SS, Drinkwater DC, Christian KG. Plastic bronchitis: is thoracic duct ligation a real surgical option? Ann Thorac Surg 2006;81(6):2281–3.

[20] Eberlein MH, Drummond MB, Haponik EF. Plastic bronchitis: a management challenge. Am J Med Sci 2008;335(2):163–9. https://doi.org/10.1097/MAJ.0b013e318068b60e.

[21] Artoni A, Selicorni A, Passamonti SM, Lecchi A, Bucciarelli P, Cerutti M, et al. Hemostatic abnormalities in Noonan syndrome. Pediatrics 2014;133(5):e1299–304. https://doi.org/10.542/peds.2013-3251.

[22] Macksey LF, White B. Anesthetic management in a pediatric patient with Noonan syndrome, mastocytosis, and von Willebrand disease: a case report. AANA J 2007;75(4):261–4.

[23] Romano AA, Allanson JE, Dahlgren J, Gelb BD, Hall B, Pierpont ME, et al. Noonan syndrome: clinical features, diagnosis, and management guidelines. Pediatrics 2010;126 (4):746–59.

[24] Jongmans MC, van der Burgt I, Hoogerbrugge PM, Noordam K, Yntema HG, Nillesen WM, et al. Cancer risk in patients with Noonan syndrome carrying a PTPN11 mutation. Eur J Hum Genet 2011;19(8):870–4. https://doi.org/10.1038/ejhg.2011.37 [Epub Mar 16].

[25] McLure HA, Yentis SM. General anaesthesia for caesarean section in a parturient with Noonan's syndrome. Br J Anaesth 1996;77(5):665–8.

[26] McBain J, Lemire EG, Campbell DC. Epidural labour analgesia in a parturient with Noonan syndrome: a case report. Can J Anaesth 2006;53(3):274–8.

[27] Hunter A, Pinsky L. An evaluation of the possible association of malignant hyperpyrexia with the Noonan syndrome using serum creatine phosphokinase levels. J Pediatr 1975;86(3):412–5.

[28] Rissam HS, Mittal SR, Wahi PL, Bidwai PS. Postoperative hyperpyrexia in a case of Noonan's syndrome. Indian Heart J 1982;34(3):180–2.

[29] King JO, Denborough MA. Anesthetic-induced malignant hyperpyrexia in children. J Pediatr 1973;83(1):37–40.

[30] Kaplan AM, Bergeson PS, Gregg SA, Curless RG. Malignant hyperthermia associated with myopathy and normal muscle enzymes. J Pediatr 1977;91(3):431–4.

[31] Lee CKCB, Hong YM, Yang SW, Lee CS, Seo JB. Spinal deformities in Noonan syndrome: a clinical review of sixty cases. J Bone Joint Surg Am 2001;83-A(10):1495–502.

[32] Croonen EA, Harmsen M, Van der Burgt I, Draaisma JM, Noordam K, Essink M, et al. Perceived motor problems in daily life: focus group interviews with people with Noonan syndrome and their relatives. Am J Med Genet A 2016;170(9):2349–56.

[33] Vegunta S, Cotugno R, Williamson A, Grebe TA. Chronic pain in Noonan syndrome: a previously unreported but common symptom. Am J Med Genet A 2015;167A (12):2998–3005. https://doi.org/10.1002/ajmg.a.37337 [Epub 2015 Aug 22].

[34] Croonen EA, Essink M, van der Burgt I, Draaisma JM, Noordam C. Nijhuis-van der Sanden MWG. Motor performance in children with Noonan syndrome. Am J Med Genet A 2017;173(9):2335–45. https://doi.org/10.1002/ajmg.a.38322 [Epub 2017 Jun 19].

[35] Reinker KA, Stevenson DA, Tsung A. Orthopaedic conditions in Ras/MAPK related disorders. J Pediatr Orthop 2011;31(5):599–605. https://doi.org/10.1097/BPO. 0b013e318220396e.

[36] Smpokou P, Tworog-Dube E, Kucherlapati RS, Roberts AE. Medical complications, clinical findings, and educational outcomes in adults with Noonan syndrome. Am J Med Genet A 2012;158A(12):3106–11. https://doi.org/10.1002/ajmg.a.35639 [Epub 2012 Nov 19].

CHAPTER 10

Oral and Dental Manifestations in Noonan Syndrome

Robert P. Anthonappa*, Nigel M. King†

*Paediatric Dentistry, Division of Oral Developmental and Behavioural Sciences, Discipline Lead and Program Convenor, UWA Dental School, The University of Western Australia, Nedlands, WA, Australia
†Faculty of Health and Medical Sciences, UWA Dental School, The University of Western Australia, Nedlands, WA, Australia

Abstract

Many oral and dental manifestations have been observed in Noonan syndrome (NS), which occur together or separately along with the general manifestations. Here, we describe the oral and dental manifestations of NS, highlighting the potential dental treatment modalities. The most commonly reported manifestations include, but are not limited to, maxillio-mandibular discrepancies, high-arched palate, micrognathia, malocclusion, anterior open-bite, posterior cross-bite, eruption disturbances, enamel defects, dental caries, eruption cysts, dilacerations, benign multiple giant cell lesions of hard and/or soft tissues, and odontogenic keratocysts and dental anomalies such as hypodontia, hyperdontia, taurodontism, microdontia, double-tooth. Therefore, it is essential that clinicians understand the nature and extent of these variations in the clinical presentation of NS patients so as to be proficient in diagnosis and the appropriate management. Furthermore, an interdisciplinary management is essential to achieve favorable treatment outcomes.

Keywords: Dental manifestations, Oral manifestations, Noonan syndrome

Abbreviations

DDE	developmental defects of enamel
DEO	demarcated enamel opacity
DIO	diffuse opacity
EH	enamel hypoplasia
EO	enamel opacity
GA	general anesthesia
MGCLs	benign multiple giant cell lesions
NS	Noonan syndrome
SRA	short-root anomaly
vWD	von Willebrand disorder

Noonan Syndrome
https://doi.org/10.1016/B978-0-12-815348-2.00009-8

INTRODUCTION

Before discussing the management of the various oral and dental manifestations that have been reported to occur in Noonan syndrome (NS), it is important to understand that a syndrome is a collection of signs and symptoms that occur in combination more frequently than would be likely by chance alone [1]. The actual features depend upon which aspects of development are affected by the abnormal genes or chromosomes. When a genetic syndrome is rare, then only single case reports are published in the literature. Consequently, in an attempt to share knowledge and information, all of the oral manifestations tend to get recorded. It is left to the future reader to determine which manifestations are specific (diagnostic) of the particular syndrome. Conversely in syndromes with a high frequency that have been repeatedly reported, recorders have refined the findings and only certain feature are considered to be of diagnostic value for that syndrome. For example, a form of cleft lip/palate, with lip pits and hypodontia, is considered to be diagnostic of Van der Woude Syndrome (Table 1).

In NS, the craniodentofacial features are well established as being characteristic of the syndrome. However, many of the oral and dental manifestations also occur in normal healthy individuals. While it is proposed to describe the dental/oral manifestations found in NS, they may, until greater quantities of data become available, be merely an association. Nevertheless, these manifestations need to be recognized and managed while being cognizant of the implication caused by the other known features of NS.

Patients commonly report oral and dental manifestations, because they impact on their functionality and ultimately the quality of life. Due to the association with an individual's general and oral health, it has been suggested that accurate early diagnosis of a condition such as NS is important [2]. Specific oral and dental manifestations that occur in NS have rarely been reported in the literature and hence are poorly recognized by healthcare providers. Several disorders with significant phenotypes overlaps with NS; such as Turner syndrome, cardiofaciocutaneous (CFC) syndrome, Costello syndrome, Leopard syndrome, Aarskog syndrome, and Baraitser-Winter syndrome [2], thus making the differential diagnosis of NS difficult and impossible from the oral manifestations. Nevertheless, the craniodentofacial structures exhibit specific features that can often aid the dental specialist in diagnosing NS. It is proposed to describe the oral and dental manifestations associated with NS, highlighting the potential treatment modalities that may be required by subjects with NS.

Table 1 List of reported oral manifestations in Noonan syndrome

Skeletal discrepancies
- Maxillo-mandibular discrepancy (Class II, Class III tendency)
- Micrognathia (small jaw)
- High-arched palate
- Anterior open bite
- Posterior cross-bite
- Malocclusion (crowding, deep-bite, and increased overjet)

Multiple giant cell lesions in the jaws or soft tissues
- Eruption cysts
- Odontogenic keratocysts

Eruption disorders
- Retained primary (deciduous) teeth
- Unerupted/impacted permanent teeth
- Premature exfoliation of primary teeth
- Infra-occluded (submerged) teeth
- Ectopic teeth
- Dilacerations

Enamel defects
- Hypoplasia

Dental anomalies
- Hypodontia (missing teeth)
- Hyperdontia (extra teeth)
- Microdontia
- Double tooth
- Taurodontism
- Short-root anomaly

Dental caries

EXTRAORAL FEATURES

The facial construct of individuals with NS includes a broad forehead, prominent eyes, hypertelorism, hooded eyelids, downslanting palpebral fissures, low-set posteriorly rotated ears with a thick helix, and a nose with a wide base and bulbous tip, thick lips, pointed chin, epicanthal folds, and ptosis. In addition, there is frequently a convex profile with an excessive vertical facial dimension (hyperdivergence) and a very recessive chin (micrognathia), see Fig. 1. In infancy, the facial appearance is characteristic and becomes subtler toward later childhood and adulthood [3]. Infants with NS usually present with a small face, which appears to be tucked beneath a large cranium, the head is large with narrowing at the temples, resulting in a tall forehead.

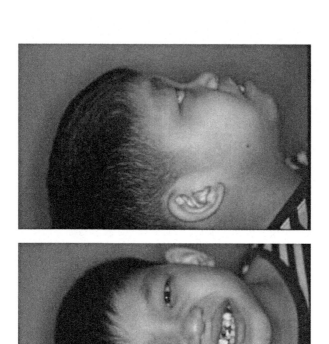

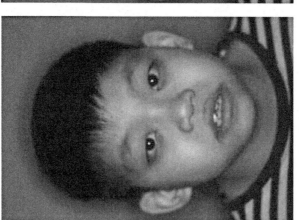

Fig. 1 Extraoral features of a patient with Noonan syndrome.

The neck is also short with a low posterior hairline. Later in childhood, the expressionless facial appearance resembles that of a myopathic face while in adolescence, the face is more triangular with a wide forehead, and pointed chin. The eyes are less prominent but have sharp features. The neck is longer than normal, and skin webbing or trapezius muscle prominence (webbed neck) is also reported to be a characteristic feature of NS [4].

INTRAORAL FEATURES

The most common dental manifestations reported to occur in to be associated with NS (Figs. 2 and 3) include severe maxillo-mandibular discrepancies, high-arched palate, tongue thrust, malocclusion, open bite and/or an increased over-jet, impacted teeth, short root length, enamel hypoplasia (EH), taurodontism,

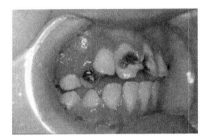 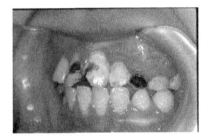

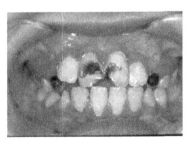

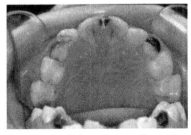 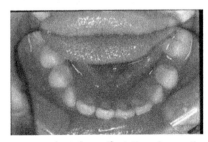

Fig. 2 Intraoral photographs illustrating the common dental manifestations in a patient with Noonan syndrome.

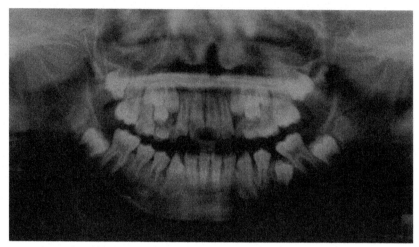

Fig. 3 Panoramic radiograph of a patient with Noonan syndrome.

dilacerations, and a range of dental anomalies including anomalies of tooth number (hypodontia, supernumerary teeth), size (microdontia), and shape (double tooth), all of which can occur in nonsyndromic individuals.

Skeletal Discrepancies

A severe discrepancy between the maxillary and mandibular arches is common. In a cohort of mutation-positive NS subjects ($N=20$), Cao et al. [5] noted a normal distribution of Class I occlusion and Class II malocclusion and a significant increased incidence of open bite (29%) and posterior cross-bite (30%) compared to the general population. Furthermore, in NS individuals, both Class II [6] and Class III [7] skeletal tendencies have been reported. An individual with a Class II skeletal relationship would exhibit a convex profile with excessive vertical facial dimension and a recessive chin, conversely, a retrognathic maxilla and prognathic mandible are evident in individuals with a Class III skeletal tendency (Fig. 4).

The maxillary dental arch is usually oval-shaped and is accompanied by a deep and constricted palatal vault [8], see Figs. 4 and 5. Affected individuals exhibit a significant tongue thrust habit (Fig. 6) and a symmetrical face with severe lip incompetence [6]—see Fig. 1. When smiling, they show the whole of the crowns of the incisor teeth and an excessive amount of gingival tissue (Fig. 1). In addition, it has been stated that NS individuals can have a

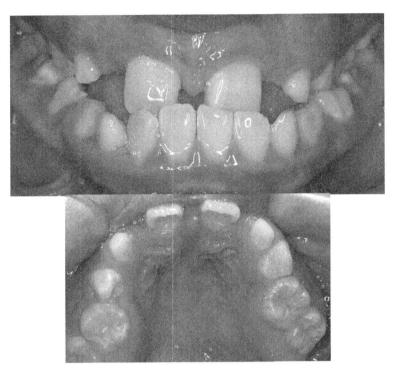

Fig. 4 Intraoral photographs showing a retrognathic maxilla and prognathic mandible in a patient with Noonan syndrome.

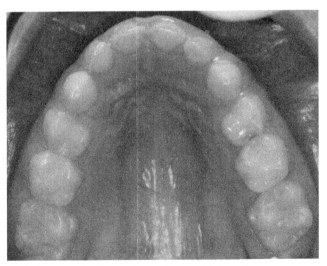

Fig. 5 Intraoral photographs illustrating a deep palatal vault.

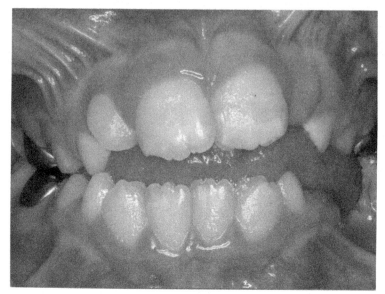

Fig. 6 Intraoral frontal photograph of a patient showing the tongue thrust habit.

moderate to severe malocclusion, anterior open-bite [9], posterior cross-bite [10], and a deep-bite [11], see Figs. 7–9. These features are often attributed to the genetic disorder and a tongue thrust habit [6]. Furthermore, the association of periodontitis with NS has been reported in two patients [12], so is bilateral enlargement of the mental foramina and inferior-alveolar canals [13].

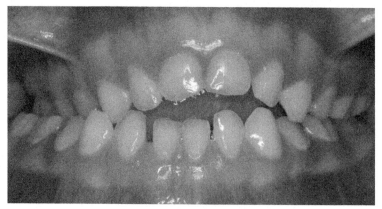

Fig. 7 Intraoral photograph of a patient showing an anterior open-bite, and a posterior cross-bite (evident on the patients right hand side).

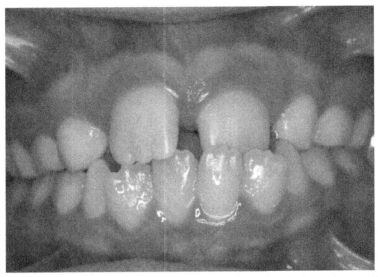

Fig. 8 Intraoral photograph of a patient showing an anterior single tooth cross-bite.

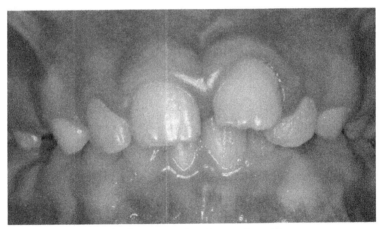

Fig. 9 Intraoral photograph of a patient showing an deep-bite.

Given the wide variation in the severity of the orthodontic problems exhibited by NS individuals, a combination of treatment approaches may be required to correct the problems that have been described earlier. These include, but are not limited to, extraction of both retained primary and/or permanent teeth, surgical removal of supernumerary teeth and/or impacted teeth, functional appliance therapy, and combined orthodontic treatment with orthognathic surgery (e.g., LeFort I impaction, mandibular advancement, and genioplasty). Regardless of the adopted treatment approach, the principle treatment objectives should always include the creation of a balanced facial profile, improved function by arranging the teeth to achieve optimal efficiency with normal overbite and overjet, and improve the health of the dentition, joints, and periodontal tissues. Given the significant growth anomalies, the ability of the clinician to obtain a good treatment outcome is heavily dependent on the level of the individual patient's cooperation.

Cherubism, a disorder characterized by abnormal bone tissue in the lower part of the face, is a finding in NS [14–16]. Most of the individuals who exhibit cherubism have few, if any, signs and symptoms affecting other parts of the body. It is usually recognized between 2 and 4 years of age, follows a variable course, and has not been reported to be related to other genetic disorders. Beginning in early childhood, both the mandible and maxilla become enlarged as the bone is replaced with painless, cyst-like growths. These growths give the cheeks a swollen, rounded appearance and often interfere with normal tooth development. Enlargement of the jaw usually continues throughout childhood and stabilizes during puberty. In some individuals, the condition may be mild and hence may remain unnoticed, while severely affected cases experience problems with vision, breathing, speech, and swallowing. In early adulthood, the abnormal growths are gradually replaced with normal bone, thus resulting in a normal facial appearance.

Although rare, benign multiple giant cell lesions (MGCLs) of the hard and/or soft tissues can develop in the craniofacial regions of NS individuals [17]. Chuong et al. [18] reported central giant cell lesions of the jaws in 2 of 17 patients with NS; while Cohen and Gorlin [19] reported of 14 cases with similar findings. Subsequently, Connor et al. [20], Dunlap et al. [15], and Betts et al. [21] reported other cases with this association. Furthermore, MGCLs are associated with jaw enlargement in 46% of affected individuals; the lesions which predominately affect the mandible have been detected between the ages of 2 and 19 years [2, 22].

Furthermore, a case of neurofibromatosis in NS with a central giant cell granuloma has been reported [23]. The giant-cell lesions are frequently found in the jaws and therefore persons with mild Noonan-like/multiple giant-cell lesion syndrome can be misdiagnosed with cherubism [24]. Pathogenic variants in *PTPN11* and *SOS1* [25] have been described in both familial and simplex cases of Noonan-like/multiple giant-cell lesion syndrome.

NS and cherubism are so essentially different that a common link is difficult to predict. However, Cohen and Gorlin [19] have proposed a syndrome, which combines patients with a phenotype of NS with MGCLs. Although it seems likely that they are independent diseases transmitted by genes closely linked on the same chromosome, this rare syndrome still requires considerable investigation to be fully delineated.

Eruption Disturbances

Tooth eruption has a strong influence on the craniofacial development; hence, eruption disturbances can be an indication of an underlying local or systemic condition. Both primary and permanent teeth have specific development sequences and timetables for eruption with age, gender, racial, and ethnic denominators. Nevertheless, a wide range of variations has been reported even in normal populations.

Occasionally, permanent incisors or premolars may erupt prematurely from these established norms, usually as a consequence of untreated dental carious lesions and/or dental traumatic injuries to the primary teeth resulting in dental abscess and possible extraction of the affected tooth. Nevertheless, eruption issues tend to cause minimum problems and are thus not extensively recorded in the literature.

In NS patients, significant delays in tooth eruption from the established norms have been reported to be more common than premature eruption. This occurs more frequently in the permanent dentition rather than in the primary dentition, although one report [10] described early exfoliation of primary canines in an NS individual. During the mixed dentition phase, all of the primary teeth are replaced by their permanent successors. Disturbances in exfoliation of the primary teeth eruption can have an influence on the permanent successor. While deviations in eruption of the maxillary incisors, canines, first permanent molars, and premolar tooth types are a frequent clinical presentation, this is largely attributed to the tooth size-arch length discrepancy [6, 11, 26]. More severe dental phenotypes have been reported, including a case report of a 13-year-old boy with multiple unerupted permanent teeth, multiple infraoccluded and retained primary teeth plus supernumerary teeth [27]. Therefore, careful monitoring of the developing permanent dentition and early diagnosis of aberrations in the exfoliation and eruption patterns are essential for timely and appropriate interventions to limit or even prevent the severity of the potential consequences.

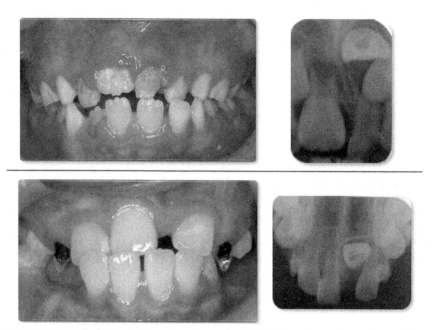

Fig. 10 Intraoral photographs and radiographs illustrating dilacerations of maxillary permanent central incisors.

Dilacerations

Dilaceration is defined as a deviation or bend in the linear relationship of a tooth crown to its root. This occurs most often in the permanent dentition and frequently affects the maxillary incisors (Fig. 10). The possible causes for dilaceration of a permanent tooth are traumatic dental injury to the primary predecessor, idiopathic developmental disturbance, a retained or ankylosed primary tooth, and the presence of supernumerary tooth or teeth. Therefore, dilacerations of permanent teeth reported in NS individuals [28] are most likely to be a coincidental occurrence rather than a true association.

Enamel Defects

Developmental defects of enamel (DDE) are defined as any alterations resulting from diverse disturbances during the process of odontogenesis (tooth formation). If they are quantitative in nature, they manifest as a deficient thickness of enamel or EH; while if they are qualitative (hypomineralization), they present as an enamel opacity (EO), either demarcated (DEO) or diffuse (DIO).

Recently, Mallineni et al. [28] reported the presence of EH in NS individuals. They found DDE on the permanent maxillary and mandibular permanent incisors in four individuals (Fig. 11). Given the high prevalence of DDE in the permanent dentition in developed countries, which is reportedly in the range of 9%–68% [29], further investigations are required to delineate the causality of DDE in individuals with NS. Nevertheless, DDE in both the primary and permanent dentitions are considered to be risk factors for dental caries (Figs. 12 and 13). Therefore, timely, appropriate intervention is strongly recommended to prevent the potential consequences of pain, dental abscess formation, and the need for extraction of the affected teeth.

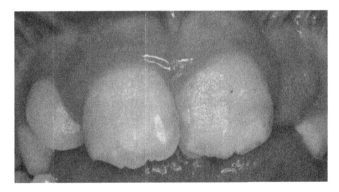

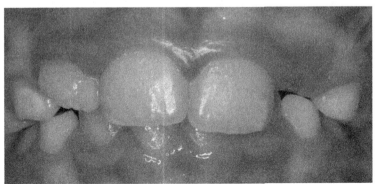

Fig. 11 Intraoral photographs showing enamel defects on the permanent maxillary incisors.

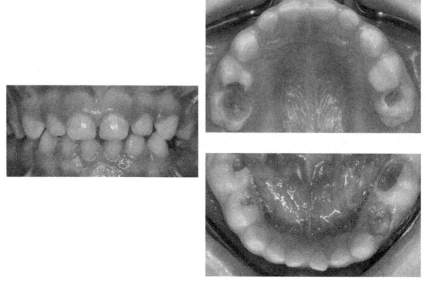

Fig. 12 Intraoral photographs of a patient showing multiple carious lesions secondary to enamel defects in the primary teeth.

Dental Anomalies
Taurodontism

A molar tooth in which the body of the tooth appears to be enlarged at the expense of the roots is said to exhibit taurodontism. It occurs in varying degrees and is classified in increasing order of severity as hypotaurodontism, mesotaurodontism, and hypertaurodontism. It can occur in both the primary as well as the permanent dentition, and is most evident in the mandibular molars [28]. Since the diagnosis of this trait can only be made reliably from a radiographic examination (Fig. 14), a sound knowledge of the associated complications is important when behavioral issues prevent the taking of radiographs. Severe clinical complications can result from the abnormal morphology of a taurodontic tooth when endodontic therapy is indicated because, the extensive length of the pulp chamber may create difficulties in locating the root canals and subsequently, in cleaning and obturation of the root canals.

Hypodontia

Hypodontia refers to the developmental absence of one or more primary or permanent teeth, excluding the third molars. The term "oligodontia" is used

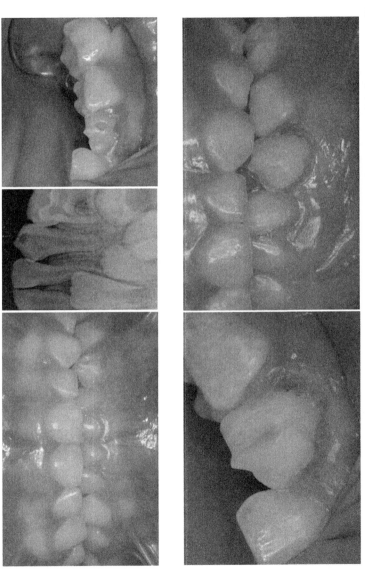

Fig. 13 Intraoral photographs and a periapical radiograph illustrating a carious lesion secondary to enamel defects in a mandibular primary canine tooth, which was restored using resin composites. *(Courtesy: Dr. Lisa Bowdin.)*

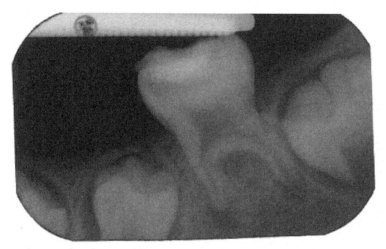

Fig. 14 Periapical radiograph showing a mandibular first permanent molar tooth exhibiting taurodontism.

for six or more missing teeth and "anodontia" for complete absence of teeth. Hypodontia is the most commonly occurring developmental dental anomaly in man and is found more often in the permanent dentition. It occurs either as an isolated abnormality or in association with several syndromes or conditions, most notably ectodermal dysplasia. The missing tooth types, namely premolars and maxillary incisors (Fig. 4), reported in NS individuals [28] are similar to the ones commonly missing in the general population [30].

Hyperdontia

Teeth in additional to the normal complement of 20 primary and 32 permanent teeth are known as supernumerary teeth. That is any tooth or structure formed from a tooth germ in excess of the usual number for any given region of the dental arch [30a]. Most supernumerary teeth occur in the premaxilla are conical-shaped, and remain unerupted due to their inverted positions [31], see Fig. 15. This is the fundamental reason why many supernumerary teeth are either unidentified or misdiagnosed. Ortega Ade et al. [32] and Toureno and Park [13] reported the occurrence of supernumerary teeth in NS individuals.

The presence of a supernumerary tooth can lead to potential complications, such as crowding of the teeth; noneruption or delayed eruption of the adjacent teeth; displacement of teeth; midline diastema; delayed exfoliation

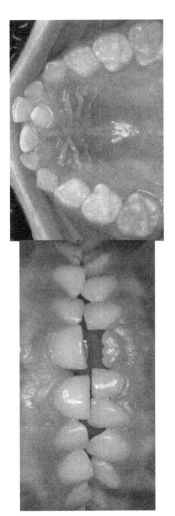
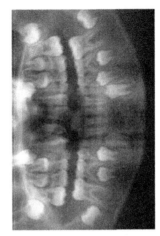
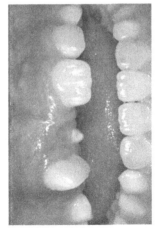

Fig. 15 Intraoral photographs and a panoramic radiograph showing supernumerary teeth in the maxillary anterior region.

of primary teeth; cyst formation; paresthesia and/or pain due to a supernumerary tooth impinging on an adjacent nerve; ectopic eruption into the nose or maxillary sinus; and compromised aesthetics. Therefore, both clinical and appropriate radiographic examinations are essential for the identification of supernumerary teeth.

Double Tooth

This anomaly is also known as fusion, germination, connation, linking tooth, and dichotomy. It is a nonspecific term used to describe any tooth-like structure resembling two complete or partially complete teeth, (Fig. 16). These teeth occur mostly in the anterior region and frequently involve the mandibular canines and the lateral incisors followed by the maxillary anterior region. The occurrence of double primary teeth involving two adjacent teeth, especially a central and lateral incisor in the maxillary arch or a lateral incisor and canine in the mandibular arch is much higher than any other type of double tooth. Because a double tooth causes aesthetic and functional problems, proper monitoring of occlusal development to prevent midline deviation, and abnormal delay of eruption of the permanent

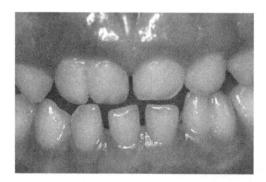

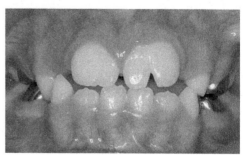

Fig. 16 Intraoral photographs showing double teeth in both the primary and permanent dentitions.

successor(s) is important. Furthermore, if a double tooth occurs in the primary dentition, it frequently serves as an indication of an anomalous number of permanent teeth in that region of the dental arch.

Short-Root Anomaly

Rhizomicry or short-root anomaly (SRA) or root dwarfism, of all permanent teeth, and resorption of both condyles has been reported by Cardiel Rios [6]. The reasons for the presence of short roots can vary from idiopathic to childhood environmental insults such as radiotherapy, chemotherapy, or dental, and systemic hereditary disorders. Both dental and systemic hereditary disorders can be associated with generalized shortness of the roots; the most probable examples of the former being dentinal dysplasia and dentinogenesis imperfecta [33], whereas the latter includes some short-stature syndromes [34]. SRA is genetically determined and orthodontic tooth movement requires changes in the orthodontic mechanics to move teeth in order to restrict damage. Orthodontic movement of teeth with SRA is contraindicated in extreme cases, only. Nevertheless, caution at all stages is required to minimize attachment loss and ensure long-term stability [35].

Dental Caries

Dental caries is an opportunistic infection caused by bacteria (in the presence of sugars), which occurs in most individuals who have different risk levels, rather than just a carious lesion. Dental caries is a global health concern and according to the World Health Organization, between 60% and 90% of school children have dental caries [36]. Recently, it has been reported that untreated dental caries in the primary dentition is the 10th most prevalent condition worldwide, affecting 621 million children [37]. Left untreated dental caries can have systemic consequences including pain, infection, swelling requiring emergency hospitalizations, and dental extractions under general anesthesia (GA). This leads to loss of school days, reduced activity, eating and sleeping difficulties, and parental distress. Consequently, the individuals' oral health-related quality of life is adversely affected.

Scientific evidence of susceptibility to dental caries in the NS populations is limited, making it difficult to establish firm conclusions. One case report, however, highlighted an equivalent or higher prevalence of caries in three individuals with NS [9]. Local risk factors determinant of caries (difficulty of access to dental care, poor dietary habits, reduced manual dexterity, poor oral hygiene, enamel defects, dental crowding, and parental neglect) override the "protective factors" (such as the buffering capacity of saliva, plus agenesis, and microdontia of the teeth) in NS individuals (Fig. 2).

Dental caries is a largely preventable condition. However, if left untreated it can lead to systemic consequences requiring emergency hospital visits and dental extractions. In addition to financial barriers preventing dental treatment access, pediatricians, nurses, the children themselves, family organizations, as well as the general dentists often overlook the early symptoms of dental caries. Therefore, delayed management can contribute to the subsequent need for complex treatment under local anesthesia, inhalation sedation, or GA. Dental treatment under GA is often the only viable option for individuals who cannot cope with the dental treatment due to their age, anxiety in the dental setting, and the invasive nature of the required treatment. The potential anesthetic problems of a patient with NS may be due to impairment of cardiopulmonary function, impaired airway, and the technical difficulties with regional anesthesia.

Antibiotic Prophylaxis

Congenital heart defects are present in 85% subjects with of NS, in whom the most prevalent cardiac anomaly is pulmonary valve stenosis, with an incidence of 50%–60% [38]. Native pulmonary valve endocarditis is an extremely rare entity in childhood and the correlation between pulmonary valve stenosis and infective endocarditis remains controversial. NS individuals with pulmonary valve stenosis are accepted as being at low risk, and antibiotic prophylaxis is no longer recommended [39]. Although pulmonary stenosis is not considered to be a common predisposing factor for infective endocarditis; it can contribute to the progression of infective endocarditis in NS patients [40]. Therefore, the need for antibiotic prophylaxis prior to dental procedures should be considered in consultation with the NS patient's cardiologist and national guidelines.

Bleeding Disorders

Between 50% and 89% of NS, subjects have a bleeding disorder. The current understanding of bleeding disorders in NS suggests four etiologies: thrombocytopenia, platelet dysfunction, von Willebrand disorder (vWD), and factor deficiencies [41]. As a significant number of NS individuals will require invasive dental procedures including dental extractions, it is important to identify which patients are at risk because of their dental procedure. Dentists need to be aware of the need to take appropriate prophylactic steps to minimize bleeding complications in NS patients. In consultation with a hematologist, an initial routine screen consisting of a complete bleeding history, platelet counts, PTT/aPTT [2], and BT [42] as well as factor XI levels [43] are recommended strategies. If any of these tests is abnormal then, when appropriate, platelet function studies, individual factor levels (II, V, VIII, IX, XI, XII), and vWD tests should be obtained [42, 43].

There is no consensus on the management of bleeding complications in patients with NS; hence, significant clinical judgment is required. The hope is that all patients have been properly screened prior to any procedure so that if abnormal bleeding does occur, the treatment can be tailored to the patient's needs. If bleeding complications of unknown etiology do occur in a patient with NS, the following is a reasonable strategy. First, use local hemostatic measures such as local anesthetics with vasoconstrictor, pressure, suture the wound, oxidized cellulose, fibrin meshes, or stomahesive tape. Subsequently, if bleeding continues, then transfer the patient to a hematology unit for further care. Furthermore, if hemostasis is achieved using local measures, review within 24 h and discuss possible omissions in the medical history including the family history of vWD, hemophilia, previous history of bleeding episodes (possible hematological undiagnosed malignancies) and refer to an hematologist for further investigations.

SUMMARY

The features of the clinical phenotypes of NS vary significantly; hence, it is important to understand the nature and extent of the phenotypic variations in affected individuals. The oral and dental manifestations of NS may occur together or separately along with the general manifestations, which have significant consequences. The most commonly reported manifestations include, but are not limited to maxillio-mandibular discrepancies, high-arched palate, micrognathia, malocclusion, anterior open-bite, posterior cross-bite, eruption disturbances, enamel defects, dental caries, eruption cysts, dilacerations, benign MGCLs of hard and/or soft tissues, and odontogenic keratocysts and dental anomalies such as hypodontia, hyperdontia, taurodontism, microdontia, and double-teeth. Therefore, it is essential that clinicians understand the nature and extent of these variations in the clinical presentation of individuals with NS so as to be proficient in facilitating the appropriate diagnosis and management. Furthermore, an interdisciplinary management is essential to achieve optimum treatment outcomes.

Oral healthcare for NS patients should commence in the first year of life and take the form of preventative measures in order to prevent subsequent problems. It is important to monitor the oral health of the patients with NS, because they are prone to severe dental caries and subsequent complex dental treatment. Prevention of early childhood caries is important so as to avoid subsequent problems during the eruption of the permanent teeth. Moreover, the identification and management of dental anomalies should be given a high priority. Finally, the timely consultation with the NS individual's physician, cardiologist, and hematologist prior to any invasive dental procedure is critical so as to identify the at-risk NS individuals and prevent any undesirable complications.

FUTURE DIRECTIONS

Oral and dental manifestations are commonly encountered in the NS patient, but to establish their true relationship to the other features of the syndrome, their prevalence and significance require further study. Most important is the determination of the relationship of dental anomalies with NS. Furthermore, the emerging relationship between the cherubism-like findings and NS should be explored to delineate the common link, if it exists between the two conditions.

REFERENCES

[1] Dorland. Dorland's illustrated medical dictionary. 32nd ed. USA: Elsevier Saunders; 2011. p. 167, ISBN: 978-1-4160-6257-8.
[2] Romano AA, Allanson JE, Dahlgren J, Gelb BD, Hall B, Pierpont ME, et al. Noonan syndrome: clinical features, diagnosis and management guidelines. Pediatrics 2010;126:746–59.
[3] Allanson JE, Hall JG, Hughes HE, Preus M, Witt RD. Noonan syndrome: hanging phenotype. Am J Med Genet 1985;21:507–14.
[4] Allanson JE. Noonan syndrome. J Med Genet 1987;24:9–13.
[5] Cao H, Alrejaye N, Klein OD, Goodwin AF, Oberoi S. A review of craniofacial and dental findings of the RASopathies. Orthod Craniofacial Res 2017;20(Suppl. 1):32–8.
[6] Cardiel Ríos SA. Correction of a severe Class II malocclusion in a patient with Noonan syndrome. Am J Orthod Dentofacial Orthop 2016;150(3):511–20. https://doi.org/10.1016/j.ajodo.2015.09.032.
[7] Asokan S, Muthu MS, Rathna Prabhu V. Noonan syndrome: a case report. J Indian Soc Pedod Prev Dent 2007;25:144–7.
[8] Nelson JF, Tsaknis PJ, Konzelman JL. Noonan's syndrome: report of a case with oral findings. J Oral Med 1978;33:94–6.
[9] Barberia Leache E, Saavedra Ontiveros D, Maroto Edo M. Etiopathogenic analysis of the caries on three patients with Noonan Syndrome. Med Oral 2003;8:136–42.

[10] Okada M, Sasaki N, Kaihara Y, Okada R, Amano H, Miura K, Kosai K. Oral findings in Noonan syndrome: report of a case. J Oral Sci 2003;45:117–21.

[11] Emral ME, Akcam MO. Noonan syndrome: a case report. J Oral Sci 2009;51:301–6.

[12] Torres-Carmona MA, Arenas-Sordo ML, Saavedra-Ontiveros D, Sánchez-Guerrero MC. Enfermedad periodontal en el síndrome de Noonan. Bol Méd Hosp Infant Mex 1991;48:271–4.

[13] Toureno L, Park JH. Atypical orofacial conditions in Noonan syndrome: a case report. J Clin Pediatr Dent 2011;36:197–202.

[14] Addante RR, Breen GH. Cherubism in a patient with Noonan's syndrome. J Oral Maxillofac Surg 1996;54:210–3.

[15] Dunlap C, Neville B, Vickers RA, O'Neil D, Barker B. The Noonan syndrome/cherubism association. Oral Surg Oral Med Oral Pathol 1989;67:698–705.

[16] Lee SM, Cooper JC. Noonan syndrome with giant cell lesions. Int J Paediatr Dent 2005;15(2):140–5.

[17] Edwards PC, Fox J, Fantasia JE, Goldberg J, Kelsch RD. Bilateral central giant cell granulomas of the mandible in an 8-year-old girl with Noonan syndrome (Noonan-like/multiple giant cell lesion syndrome). Oral Surg Oral Med Oral Pathol Oral Radiol Endod 2005;99:334–40.

[18] Chuong R, Kaban LB, Kozakewich H, Perez-Atayde A. Central giant cell lesions of the jaws: a clinicopathologic study. J Oral Maxillofac Surg 1986;44:708–13.

[19] Cohen Jr. MM, Gorlin RJ. Noonan-like/multiple giant cell lesion syndrome. Am J Med Genet 1991;40:159–66.

[20] Connor JM, Evans DA, Goose DH. Multiple odontogenic keratocysts in a case of the Noonan syndrome. Br J Oral Surg 1982;20(3):213–6.

[21] Betts NJ, Stewart JC, Fonseca RJ, Scott RF. Multiple central giant cell lesions with a Noonan-like phenotype. Oral Surg Oral Med Oral Pathol 1993;76(5):601–7.

[22] Karbach J, Coerdt W, Wagner W, Bartsch O. Case report: Noonan syndrome with multiple giant cell lesions and review of the literature. Am J Med Genet A 2012;158A(9):2283–9.

[23] Yazdizadeh M, Tapia JL, Baharvand M, Radfar L. A case of neurofibromatosis-Noonan syndrome with a central giant cell granuloma. Oral Surg Oral Med Oral Pathol Oral Radiol Endod 2004;98:316–20.

[24] Jafarov T, Ferimazova N, Reichenberger E. Noonan-like syndrome mutations in PTPN11 in patients diagnosed with cherubism. Clin Genet 2005;68(2):190–1.

[25] Hanna N, Parfait B, Talaat IM, Vidaud M, Elsedfy HH. SOS1: a new player in the Noonan-like/multiple giant cell lesion syndrome. Clin Genet 2009;75(6):568–71.

[26] Sahebjamee M, Ameri NG, Farhud DD. First report of new oral findings in a case with Noonan syndrome. Iranian J Publ Health 2008;37:131–7.

[27] Uloopi KS, Madhuri V, Gopal AS, Vinay C, Chandrasekhar R. Multiple unerupted permanent teeth associated with Noonan syndrome. Ann Med Health Sci Res 2015;5(4):317–20. https://doi.org/10.4103/2141-9248.160190.

[28] Mallineni SK, Yung Yiu CK, King NM. Oral manifestations of Noonan syndrome: review of the literature and a report of four cases. Rom J Morphol Embryol 2014;55(4):1503–9.

[29] Anthonappa RP, King NM. Enamel defects in the permanent dentition: prevalence and etiology. In: Planning and care for children and adolescents with dental enamel defects. 2015 ed., vol. 15. London: Springer; 2015. p. 15–30.

[30] Polder BJ, Van't Hof MA, Van der Linden FP, Kuijpers-Jagtman AM. A meta-analysis of the prevalence of dental agenesis of permanent teeth. Community Dent Oral Epidemiol 2004;32(3):217–26.

[30a] Omer RS, Anthonappa RP, King NM. Determination of the optimum time for surgical removal of unerupted anterior supernumerary teeth. Pediatr Dent 2010;32(1):14–20.

[31] Anthonappa RP, King NM, Rabie AB. Prevalence of supernumerary teeth based on panoramic radiographs revisited. Pediatr Dent 2013;35(3):257–61.

[32] Ortega Ade O, Guaré Rde O, Kawaji NS, Ciamponi AL. Orofacial aspects in Noonan syndrome: 2 case report. J Dent Child 2008;75:85–90.

[33] Apajalahti S, Arte S, Pirinen S. Short root anomaly in families and its association with other dental anomalies. Eur J Oral Sci 1999;107:97–101.

[34] Apajalahti S, Höltta P, Turtola L, Pirinen S. Prevalence of short-root anomaly in healthy young adults. Acta Odontol Scand 2002;60:56–9.

[35] Valladares Neto J, Rino Neto J, de Paiva JB. Orthodontic movement of teeth with short root anomaly: should it be avoided, faced or ignored? Dental Press J Orthod 2013;18 (6):72–85.

[36] World Health Organisation. Oral health World Health Organisation, http://www. who.int/mediacentre/factsheets/fs318/en/; 2012. Accessed 8 January 2017.

[37] Kassebaum NJ, Bernabe E, Dahiya M, Bhandari B, Murray CJ, Marcenes W. Global burden of untreated caries: a systematic review and metaregression. J Dent Res 2015;94(5):650–8.

[38] Sznajer Y, Keren B, Baumann C, Pereira S, Alberti C, Elion J, et al. The spectrum of cardiac anomalies in Noonan syndrome as a result of mutations in the PTPN11 gene. Pediatrics 2007;119(6):e1325–31.

[39] Nishimura RA, Carabello BA, Faxon DP, Freed MD, Lytle BW, O'Gara PT, et al. ACC/AHA 2008 guideline update on valvular heart disease: focused update on infective endocarditis: a report of the American College of Cardiology/American Heart Association Task Force on Practice Guidelines endorsed by the Society of Cardiovascular Anesthesiologists, Society for Cardiovascular Angiography and Interventions, and Society of Thoracic Surgeons. J Am Coll Cardiol 2008;52(8):676–85.

[40] Hatemi AC, Gursoy M, Tongut A, Bicakhan B, Guzeltas A, Cetin G, Kansiz E. Pulmonary stenosis as a predisposing factor for infective endocarditis in a patient with Noonan syndrome. Tex Heart Inst J 2010;37(1):99–101.

[41] Briggs BJ, Dickerman JD. Bleeding disorders in Noonan syndrome. Pediatr Blood Cancer 2012;58(2):167–72.

[42] Staudt JM, Van Der Horst CMAM, Peters M, et al. Bleeding diathesis in Noonan syndrome. Scand J Plast Reconstr Surg Hand Surg 2005;39:247–8.

[43] Singer ST, Hurst D, Addiego JE. Bleeding disorders in Noonan syndrome: three case reports and review of the literature. J Pediatr Hematol Oncol 1997;19:130–4.

FURTHER READING

[44] Bufalino A, Carrera M, Carlos R, Coletta RD. Giant cell lesions in Noonan syndrome: case report and review of the literature. Head Neck Pathol 2010;4:174–7.

[45] Cancino CMH, Gaiao L, Sant'Ana Filho M, Oliveira FAM. Giant cell lesions with a Noonan-like phenotype: a case report. J Contemp Dent Pract 2007;8:67–73.

[46] Lerardo G, Luzzi V, Panetta F, Sfasciotti GL, Polimeni A. Noonan syndrome: a case report. Eur J Paediatr Dent 2010;11:97–100.

[47] Lucker GP, Steijlen PM. Widespread leucokeratosis in Noonan's syndrome. Clin Exp Dermatol 1994;19:414–7.

[48] Sugar A, Ezsias A, Bloom AL, Morcos WE. Orthognathic surgery in a patient with Noonan syndrome. J Oral Maxillofac Surg 1994;52:421–5.

Management of Noonan Syndrome

A Clinical Guideline

Noonan Syndrome Guideline Development Group

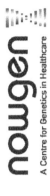

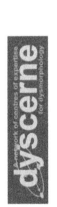

Contents

Introduction

Introduction...

... to Noonan Syndrome (NS)

Noonan syndrome (NS) is one of the more common genetic conditions.

The incidence of NS is estimated as 1 in 1,000 to 1 in 2,500 births, so it is still a relatively rare condition.

The severity of NS is the same in males and females.

The main features are congenital heart defects, short stature and characteristic facial features.

Early motor delay associated with hypotonia is not necessarily associated with later learning difficulty, and most adults with NS are able to lead independent autonomous lives.

... to the Noonan Syndrome Guideline Development Project

The guidelines have been developed using a robust methodology based on the one utilised by the Scottish Intercollegiate Guidelines Network (SIGN). The method has been adapted to suit rare conditions where the evidence base is limited, and where expert consensus plays a greater role. The members of the guideline development group are listed on page 30.

... to the Noonan Syndrome Clinical Management Guidelines

What are the aims of the guidelines?

The guidelines aim to provide clear and wherever possible, evidence-based recommendations for the management of patients with Noonan syndrome.

Who are they aimed at?

These guidelines are provided for people with NS to use with their primary care and specialist clinicians as many healthcare professionals will not have had personal experience of managing Noonan syndrome. As it is a multisystem disorder, people with NS may require various tests, screening, assessments, referrals and multidisciplinary interventions at different stages of their lives. These guidelines lay out these requirements in a clear format that is accessible to anybody who is involved in the care of an individual with NS.

How are they organised?

The guidelines are divided into recommendations for four age groups:

- Neonatal and Infancy—0–1 years old   - Childhood: 1–11 years old   - Adolescence: 11–18 years old   - Adulthood: 18 years old +

Page 4 contains an overview of the diagnostic criteria and clinical features of NS, and page 5 lists the suggested baseline investigations. Subsequently, the guidelines are organised into specific age groups. For each group, management issues along with any recommended tests/screenings are listed, and follow-up options depending on the outcome of the test or screening are indicated.

NB. ABNL= Abnormal

A full list of references starts on page 19, organised by body system, which can be used as a signpost to further information on specific aspects of NS for healthcare professionals.

Additionally, there is a list of useful contacts for parents and families affected by NS, on page 29.

Diagnosis and clinical features of Noonan Syndrome

Diagnostic features of NS (van der Burgt 1997)

Feature	A = Major	B = Minor
1. Facial	Typical face (Facial features of NS vary over time and may have only subtle differences. Expert assessment is therefore Required. See Allanson 1987—full reference p.19).	Suggestive face
2. Cardiac	Pulmonary valve stenosis and/or hypertrophic cardiomyopathy (HCM)	Other cardiac defect
3. Height	< 3th centile	< 10th centile
4. Chest wall	Pectus carinatum/excavatum	Broad thorax
5. Family History	First degree relative with definite NS	First degree relative suggestive of NS
6. Other	Mild developmental delay, cryptorchidism AND lymphatic dysplasia	Mild developmental delay, cryptorchidism, OR lymphatic dysplasia

Definitive NS:

Criterion 1A +			Criterion 1B +	
One of 2A–6A	Two of 2B–6B	Two of 2A–6A	Two of 2A–6A	Three of 2B–6B

*Currently, mutation testing will prove a diagnosis of Noonan Syndrome in 70% of cases; in 30% the responsible gene remains unknown.

The diagnosis of NS should be considered in parents when a child is diagnosed with the syndrome.

Given the number of different genes where mutations can cause NS, the appropriateness and sequence of gene testing should be decided by a clinical geneticist.

Differential diagnoses:

- Cardio-facio-cutaneous syndrome (CFC)
- Costello syndrome
- LEOPARD syndrome
- King-Denborough Syndrome (phenotypically distinct. Malignant hyperthermia is not described in NS)

NB–Neurofibromatosis-Noonan syndrome formed part of the differential diagnosis in the past; it is now known that some patients with either of these conditions will have overlapping clinical features, due to the causative mutations occurring in the same biological pathway.

Recommended baseline investigations in Noonan Syndrome

Noonan Syndrome Clinical Management Guidelines

Clinical Features of Noonan Syndrome

(where an investigation is not indicated for a specific clinical feature, please refer to the relevant age group-specific page for management recommendations)

- Congenital heart defects (e.g. pulmonary stenosis, hypertrophic cardiomyopathy, atrial septal defect)
- Failure to thrive/slow growth rate/feeding problems
- Short stature
- Developmental delay and neuropsychological/behavioural issues
- Minor renal anomalies
- Bleeding disorders
- Visual problems (e.g. posterior segment ocular changes and anterior segment ocular abnormalities)

Baseline investigations

- Full cardiac evaluation at diagnosis.
- Monitor and plot growth on appropriate NS and age-based growth chart.
- Refer patient in second half of first year or at diagnosis for formal developmental assessment.
- Baseline neuropsychological assessment at primary school entry.
- Refer for renal ultrasound at diagnosis.
- Carry out baseline coagulation screening in patients aged 5+, or earlier if major procedure to be undertaken. (Prothrombin Time (PT) Activated Partial Thromboplastin Time (aPPT) and FXI assay.)
- Refer for specialist ophthalmology assessment at the point of diagnosis.

Recommendations for the management of Noonan Syndrome
~ in neonates & infancy (1) ~

Recommended Testing/Screening		Clinical Management Recommendations
• Feeding assessment		Refer for dietary assessment and evaluation of swallowing if needed.
	ABNL	Refer to speech therapist for management if necessary.
	ABNL	Frequent vomiting should prompt investigation for gastro-oesophageal reflux and malrotation.
	ABNL	Treat with anti-reflux measures. Persistent vomiting or food refusal may require tube feeding (although this is rare).
• Full cardiac evaluation		At diagnosis.
	ABNL	If hypertrophic cardiomyopathy (HCM) is found, follow up carefully. Management of congenital heart disease is as per the general population, however a dysplastic valve is more likely and therefore surgery may be more likely to be necessary.
• Growth monitoring		Measure height, weight and occipitofrontal circumference (OFC) at birth and 1-3 monthly. Plot on NS-specific growth charts.
	ABNL	Routine paediatric investigations for failure to thrive and reduced growth velocity.
• Neuropsychological and Behavioural Issues	ABNL	Refer for formal developmental assessment in 2nd half of first year.
	ABNL	Developmental delay caused by hypotonia will improve with occupational and physiotherapy. Management of developmental delay will be as per the general population.
• Neurology–potential complications in NS include seizures, craniosynostosis, hydrocephalus and Arnold Chiari Malformation.		Low threshold for investigation of neurological symptoms e.g. consider Arnold-Chiari malformation and hydrocephalus if patient presents with headache or other neurological symptoms, and refer for MRI if suspected.
• Renal ultrasound	ABNL	Refer to paediatric nephrologist for management if renal anomalies are identified in ultrasound at diagnosis.

Noonan Syndrome Clinical Management Guidelines

Recommendations for the management of Noonan Syndrome

~ in neonates & infancy (2) ~

Recommended Testing/Screening		Clinical Management Recommendations
• Coagulation screening		To be carried out before any major surgery in neonates/infants, and at least once during childhood.
• Check for cryptorchidism	ABNL	Manage in the standard way at the appropriate time.
• Skin problems: Keratosis Pilaris/Ulerythema		Avoid skin dryness, which can be worsened by long hot baths, perfumed soaps and dry atmospheres.
	ABNL	Manage using emollients, keratolytic agents e.g. salicylic acid in urea cream, if tolerated, or short courses of topical steroids if necessary (especially if erythematous). Within a specialist dermatology setting, it should be noted that retinoids may not be a first choice treatment as they have been shown not to work in some NS patients.
• Genetic mutation screening		Should be considered in the context of genetic management—which genes are tested for should be decided by a clinical geneticist.
• Vision screening: squint, posterior segment ocular changes and anterior segment ocular abnormalities have been described in NS.	ABNL	Refer for baseline evaluation at point of diagnosis.
		Ophthalmic follow up/management as deemed appropriate by the ophthalmologist.
• Hearing assessment		Refer for baseline evaluation in 2nd half of first year.
	ABNL	Management in standard way.

! Anaesthesia

NS can cause coagulation difficulties that should be evaluated prior to surgical procedures so that care, including anaesthesia, can be planned accordingly.
Patients with NS and haemodynamically significant cardiac involvement such as severe hypertrophic cardiomyopathy need to treated according to the usual principles for patients with such cardiovascular risk factors.
Patients with NS may have craniofacial and/or vertebral anomalies that could affect intubation or the administration of spinal anaesthesia.

Recommendations for the management of Noonan Syndrome
~ in childhood (1) ~

Recommended Testing/Screening		Clinical Management Recommendations
• Echocardiogram (ECHO)		Annually until the age of 3 and then at 5 and 10 years old, to assess for onset of HCM.
	ABNL	If results indicate HCM, follow-up regularly.
		Management of congenital heart disease is as per the general population, however a dysplastic valve is more likely and surgery may be more likely to be necessary.
		If ECHO results are normal at the age of 10 years old and older, cardiac follow up remains necessary due to the ongoing increased risk of cardiomyopathy.
• Growth assessment		Nearly half of children with NS will reach a height within the normal range without growth hormone (GH) intervention.
		Modest response to growth hormone therapy (GHT) has been documented but some NS patients will continue to grow into their late teens/early twenties (because of late puberty) and thereby reach normal range.
		Final height may also be influenced by parental height.
		Plot growth on NS growth charts.
	ABNL	All children with a height below the mean for NS should be referred to a paediatric endocrinologist for assessment.
Growth hormone (GH) axis evaluation	**ABNL**	If height is below 2.5 standard deviations (SD) from the mean on standard childhood charts, GHT may be considered without evaluation of the GH axis.
		If IGF-1 levels are low, testing of the GH axis should be considered to show growth hormone deficiency (GHD).
GH & hypertrophic cardiomyopathy (HCM)		**NB.** While many consider existing HCM or malignancy as relative contraindications to GHT, there are no data to support this claim.
		Additionally, there is no evidence of an increased risk of HCM or malignancy developing in people with NS undertaking GHT.
• Coagulation screening		Should be carried out at least once during mid/late childhood (5—11 years old), and before major surgery.
	ABNL	Aspirin should be withheld before any surgical interventions, as per standard practice.

Recommendations for the management of Noonan Syndrome
~ in childhood (2) ~

Recommended Testing/Screening		Clinical Management Recommendations
• **Neuropsychological and Behavioural Issues:** hypotonia and motor delay are common in NS and can cause developmental delay.		Screening for developmental delay and full neuropsychological assessment at primary (to include speech acquisition) and secondary school entry, and if/when symptomatic.
		Assess intellectual/cognitive abilities with special attention for learning difficulties as a result of motor delay, executive dysfunctions and inattention.
	ABNL	Developmental delay caused by hypotonia will improve with occupational and physiotherapy.
		Referral for speech therapy if acquisition is delayed.
		Management of developmental delay will be as per the general population.
		Ongoing review and support of learning and development with further assessment of special educational needs as required.
• **Neurology**—potential complications in NS include seizures, craniosynostosis, hydrocephalus and Arnold Chiari Malformation.		Low threshold for investigation of neurological symptoms e.g. consider Arnold-Chiari malformation and hydrocephalus if patient presents with headache or other neurological symptoms, and refer for MRI if suspected.
• **Musculoskeletal**	ABNL	Monitor for scoliosis. Be aware that it can worsen with GHT.
	ABNL	Talipes occurs in 5 % of NS patients and should be managed as per the general population.
	ABNL	Refer for occupational therapy for management of hypermobility.
• **Feeding assessment:** if necessary—most feeding issues will have resolved by 18 months.	ABNL	Refer for dietary assessment and evaluation of swallowing if needed.
		Refer to speech therapist for management if necessary.
	ABNL	Frequent vomiting should prompt investigation for gastro-oesophageal reflux and malrotation.
		Treat with anti-reflux measures. Persistent vomiting or food refusal may require tube feeding (although this is rare).
• **Check for cryptorchidism**	ABNL	Manage in the standard way at the appropriate time.
• **Lymphoedema:** There is an increased risk of developing lymphoedema in NS, throughout childhood and later life.	ABNL	Management should be the same as for general population.

Recommendations for the management of Noonan Syndrome
~ in childhood (3) ~

Recommended Testing/Screening

- **Skin problems:**
  Keratosis Pilaris/Ulerythema

- **Vision screening:** squint, posterior segment ocular changes and anterior segment ocular abnormalities are frequent in NS.

- **Hearing assessments:** NS patients have an increased risk of conductive hearing loss. Sensorineural hearing loss is rare but has been described.

- **Dental screening**

  Giant cell lesions of the jaw

Clinical Management Recommendations

Avoid skin dryness, which can be worsened by long hot baths, perfumed soaps and dry atmospheres.

ABNL Manage using emollients, keratolytic agents e.g. salicylic acid in urea cream, if tolerated, or short courses of topical steroids if necessary (especially if erythematous).
Within a specialist dermatology setting, it should be noted that retinoids may not be a first choice treatment as they have been shown not to work in some NS patients.

Unless already under ophthalmic management, NS patients should be referred to an ophthalmologist for assessment if/as appropriate.

Monitor hearing annually from 1—11 years old to prevent speech development problems.

Published evidence on the management of routine dental problems in NS is limited. Enrol patient in an individualised preventative oral healthcare programme from an early age.

ABNL Routine follow up and regular dental examinations by a family dentist or local community dental services are essential.
Missing teeth/malocclusion/other dental anomalies: refer to a consultant in paediatric dentistry for multidisciplinary management.

ABNL Refer to Oral/Maxillofacial/Head & Neck Surgeon or expert dental care centre.

! Anaesthesia
NS can cause coagulation difficulties that should be evaluated prior to surgical procedures so that care, including anaesthesia, can be planned accordingly.
Patients with NS and haemodynamically significant cardiac involvement such as severe hypertrophic cardiomyopathy need to treated according to the usual principles for patients with such cardiovascular risk factors.
Patients with NS may have craniofacial and/or vertebral anomalies that could affect intubation or the administration of spinal anaesthesia.

Recommendations for the management of Noonan Syndrome
~ in adolescence (1) ~

Recommended Testing/Screening	Clinical Management Recommendations
• Echocardiogram (ECHO)	An ECHO in adolescence is recommended as this is when familial HCM may first be identified.
	Continued cardiac follow up throughout adolescence is important.
• Puberty	The likelihood of delayed puberty should be anticipated, and appropriate education and counselling provided around this issue.
• Neuropsychological and Behavioural Issues	Access to social skills training, and programmes to teach basic self help and daily living skills, if required.
	Screen for mood and anxiety disorders if suspected.
	[ABNL] If necessary, consider pharmacological management.
• Neurology—potential complications in NS include seizures, craniosynostosis, hydrocephalus and Arnold Chiari malformation)	No routine screening is recommended, however there should be a low threshold for investigation of neurological symptoms e.g. consider Arnold-Chiari malformation and hydrocephalus if patient presents with headache or other neurological symptoms, and refer for MRI if suspected.
	[ABNL] Management of specific complications, including epilepsy, will be as per the general population.
• Coagulation screening	Screen before any surgical intervention, and withhold aspirin prior to surgery, as per standard practice.
• Musculoskeletal	Monitor for scoliosis.
	Be aware that scoliosis can worsen with GHT and in adolescence.
• Thyroid screening	Screen blood for thyroid abnormalities every 3—5 years in older children and adults.
	[ABNL] Manage anomalies as in general population.
• Lymphoedema	There is an increased risk of developing lymphoedema in NS, throughout childhood and later life.
	[ABNL] Management should be the same as for general population.

11

Recommendations for the management of Noonan Syndrome
~ in adolescence (2) ~

Recommended Testing/Screening

- **Skin problems:**
  Keratosis Pilaris/Ulerythema

- **Vision screening:** squint, posterior segment ocular changes and anterior segment ocular abnormalities have been described in NS.

- **Dental screening**

  Giant cell lesions of the jaw

- **Genetic counselling**

Clinical Management Recommendations

Avoid skin dryness, which can be worsened by long hot baths, perfumed soaps and dry atmospheres.
ABNL Manage using emollients, keratolytic agents e.g. salicylic acid in urea cream, if tolerated, or short courses of topical steroids if necessary (especially if erythematous).
Within a specialist dermatology setting, it should be noted that retinoids may not be a first choice treatment as they have been shown not to work in some NS patients.

Unless already under ophthalmic management, NS patients should be referred to an ophthalmologist for assessment if/as appropriate.

Published evidence on the management of routine dental problems in NS is limited. Routine follow up and regular dental examinations by a family dentist or local community dental services are essential.
ABNL Missing teeth/malocclusion/other dental anomalies: refer to a consultant in paediatric dentistry for multidisciplinary management.
ABNL Refer to Oral/Maxillofacial/Head & Neck Surgeon or expert dental care centre.

Refer for genetic counselling, mutation testing and discussion of risks to children and options in pregnancy, at an appropriate time.

! Anaesthesia
NS can cause coagulation difficulties that should be evaluated prior to surgical procedures so that care, including anaesthesia, can be planned accordingly.
Patients with NS and haemodynamically significant cardiac involvement such as severe hypertrophic cardiomyopathy need to treated according to the usual principles for patients with such cardiovascular risk factors.
Patients with NS may have craniofacial and/or vertebral anomalies that could affect intubation or the administration of spinal anaesthesia.

Recommendations for the management of Noonan Syndrome
~ in adulthood (1) ~

Recommended Testing/Screening	Clinical Management Recommendations
• Genetic counselling	Refer for genetic counselling, mutation testing and discussion of risks to children and options in pregnancy.
• Fertility issues	Care providers should be made aware of the increased risk of infertility in males with NS, and not just in those with cryptorchidism. Refer to a fertility clinic or endocrinologist if necessary.
• In pregnancy — Fetal considerations	Prenatal features include; polyhydramnios, increased nuchal translucency, hydrops fetalis and cystic hygroma, with or without associated ascites, pleural effusion, renal abnormalities and congenital heart defects. Chorionic villus sampling (CVS) or amniocentesis is possible—referral to a clinical genetics service preconceptually is ideal— if parental mutation is known and couple wish for a prenatal diagnosis.
— Maternal considerations	Ultrasounds at 12—14 and 20 weeks and undertake mutation analysis if parental mutation known and clinical features are suggestive, if required. Potential difficulties, for example those arising from coagulation defects during childbirth, should be considered and planned for as appropriate.
• Neuropsychological and Behavioural Issues	Repeat neuropsychological assessment if patient is symptomatic of mood/anxiety disorder(s), or if cognitive impairments are suspected. Pay extra attention to the evaluation of social cognition and social embedding. Consider the risk of under-diagnosing because of problems in expressing emotions. If necessary, consider pharmacological management. Facilitate access to support for employment, self help and independent living. Social skills intervention as needed.
• Neurology–potential complications in NS include seizures, craniosynostosis, hydrocephalus and Arnold Chiari malformation)	Low threshold for investigation of neurological symptoms e.g. consider Arnold-Chiari malformation and hydrocephalus if patient presents with headache or other neurological symptoms, and refer for MRI if suspected. Management of specific complications, including epilepsy, will be as per the general population.
• Coagulation screening	Screen before any surgical intervention, and withhold aspirin prior to surgery, as per standard practice.
• Cardiac screening	Newly diagnosed adults: full cardiac evaluation including ECHO. Previously diagnosed adults: regular cardiac assessment of existing heart disease, or cardiac evaluation incase aortic disease missed previously.
Pulmonary artery intervention	Follow up for pulmonary valve insufficiency.

ABNL (Fetal considerations)
ABNL (Neuropsychological and Behavioural Issues)
ABNL (Neurology)

Recommendations for the management of Noonan Syndrome
~ in adulthood (2) ~

Recommended Testing/Screening	Clinical Management Recommendations
• **Thyroid screening**	Screen blood for thyroid abnormalities every 3—5 years.
	(ABNL) Manage anomalies as in general population.
• **Lymphoedema**	There is an increased risk of developing lymphoedema in NS, throughout adulthood.
	(ABNL) Management should be the same as for general population.
• **Skin problems:** Keratosis Pilaris/Ulerythema	Avoid skin dryness, which can be worsened by long hot baths, perfumed soaps and dry atmospheres.
	(ABNL) Manage using emollients, keratolytic agents e.g. salicylic acid in urea cream, if tolerated, or short courses of topical steroids if necessary (especially if erythematous).
	Within a specialist dermatology setting, it should be noted that retinoids may not be a first choice treatment as they have been shown not to work in some NS patients.
• **Vision screening:** squint, posterior segment ocular changes and anterior segment ocular abnormalities have been described in NS.	Unless already under ophthalmic management, NS patients should be referred to an ophthalmologist for assessment if/as appropriate.
• **Dental screening**	Published evidence on the management of routine dental problems in NS is limited.
	Routine follow up and regular dental examinations by a family dentist or local community dental services are essential.
	(ABNL) Missing teeth/malocclusion/other dental anomalies: refer to a consultant in dentistry for multidisciplinary management.
Giant cell lesions of the jaw	*(ABNL)* Refer to Oral/Maxillofacial/Head & Neck Surgeon or expert dental care centre.

! Anaesthesia

NS can cause coagulation difficulties that should be evaluated prior to surgical procedures so that care, including anaesthesia, can be planned accordingly.
Patients with NS and haemodynamically significant cardiac involvement such as severe hypertrophic cardiomyopathy need to treated according to the usual principles for patients with such cardiovascular risk factors.
Patients with NS may have craniofacial and/or vertebral anomalies that could affect intubation or the administration of spinal anaesthesia.

Noonan Syndrome Clinical Management Guidelines

NOONAN SYNDROME BOYS
Birth to 36 Months
Length for Age and Weight for Length*

Name: _____

DOB: _____ ID: _____

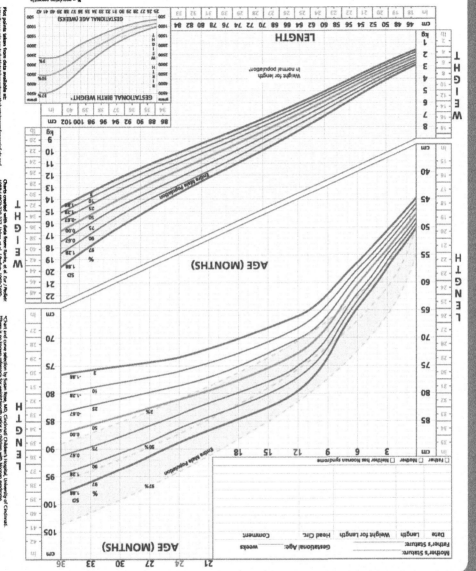

Novo Nordisk Inc.
100 College Road West
Princeton, New Jersey 08540 U.S.A.
© 2007 Novo Nordisk Inc.
13254 1A June 2007 Printed in the U.S.A.

% = population percentile   SD = standard deviation

NOONAN SYNDROME GIRLS
Birth to 36 Months
Length for Age and Weight for Length*

Name: _____

DOB: _____ ID: _____

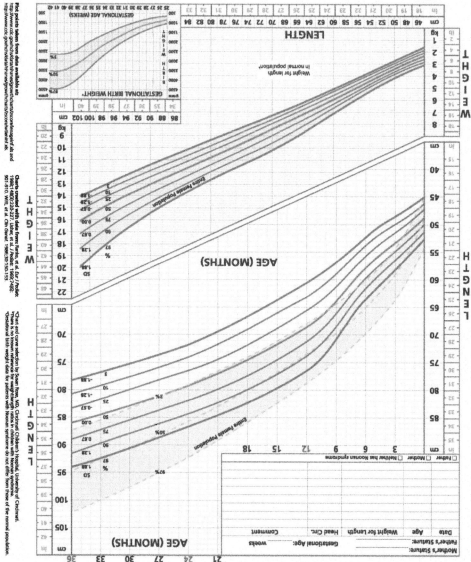

novo nordisk

Novo Nordisk Inc.
100 College Road West
Princeton, New Jersey 08540 U.S.A.

© 2007 Novo Nordisk Inc.
132541C June 2007 Printed in the U.S.A.

% = population percentile
SD = standard deviation

Plot points taken from data available at:
http://www.cdc.gov/nchs/data/nhanes/growthcharts/zscore/lenageinf.xls and
http://www.cdc.gov/nchs/data/nhanes/growthcharts/zscore/wtleninf.xls.

Charts created with data from: Ranke, et al. Eur J Pediatr.
1988;148(3):220-227. Usher, et al. J Pediatr. 1969;74(6):
901-910. Witt, et al. Clin Genet. 1986;30:150-153.

Chart and curve selection by Susan Rose, MD, Cincinnati Children's Hospital, University of Cincinnati.
*Chart and curve selection by Susan Rose, MD, Cincinnati Children's Hospital, University of Cincinnati.
*There is no known reference for weight/length ratios in children with Noonan syndrome.
*Gestational birth weight data for patients with Noonan syndrome do not differ from those of the normal population.

Noonan Syndrome Clinical Management Guidelines

NOONAN SYNDROME BOYS
2 to 20 Years
Stature and Growth Velocity for Age[a]

Name: _____

DOB: _____ ID: _____

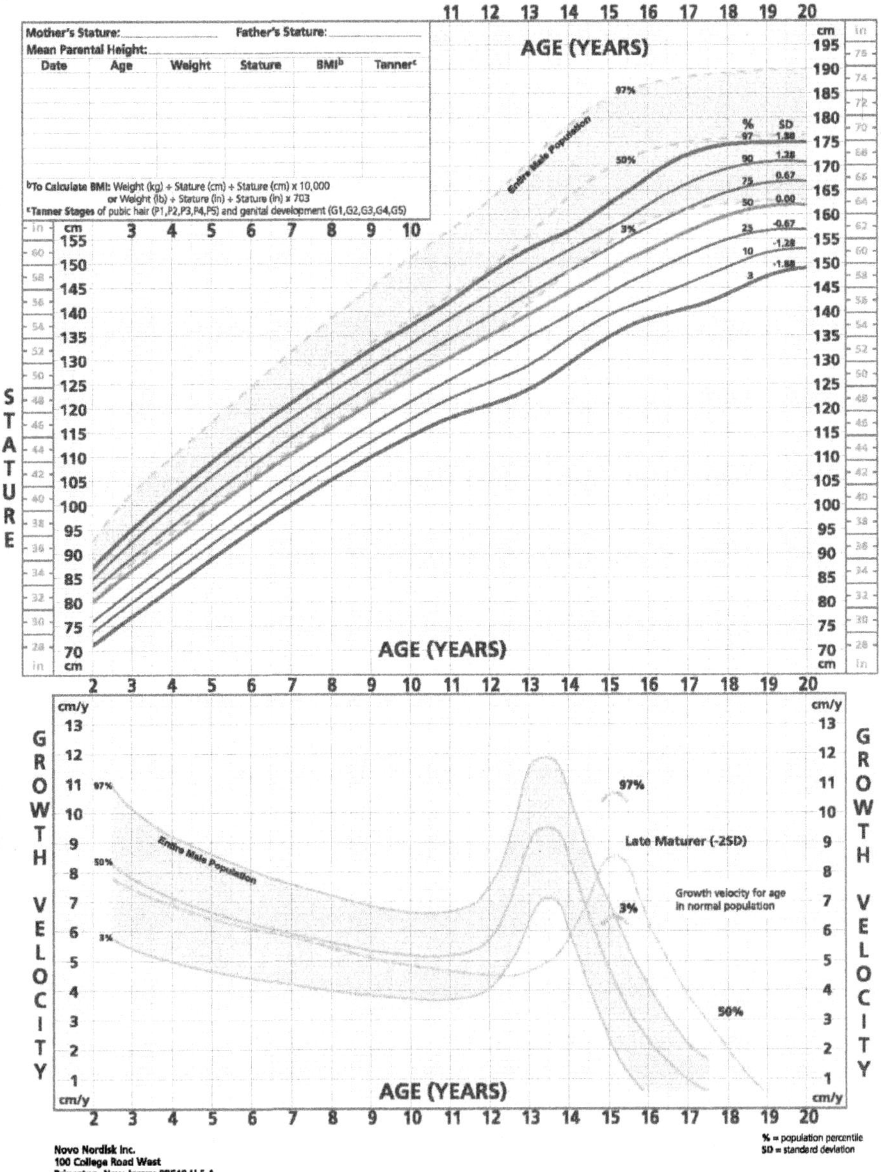

Mother's Stature: _____ Father's Stature: _____
Mean Parental Height: _____

Date	Age	Weight	Stature	BMI[b]	Tanner[c]

[b] To Calculate BMI: Weight (kg) ÷ Stature (cm) ÷ Stature (cm) × 10,000
or Weight (lb) ÷ Stature (in) ÷ Stature (in) × 703
[c] Tanner Stages of pubic hair (P1,P2,P3,P4,P5) and genital development (G1,G2,G3,G4,G5)

AGE (YEARS)

STATURE

GROWTH VELOCITY

AGE (YEARS)

% = population percentile
SD = standard deviation

Novo Nordisk Inc.
100 College Road West
Princeton, New Jersey 08540 U.S.A.

© 2007 Novo Nordisk Inc.
1325418 June 2007 Printed in the U.S.A.

Noonan Syndrome Clinical Management Guidelines

NOONAN SYNDROME GIRLS
2 to 20 Years
Stature and Growth Velocity for Age*

Name: _____
DOB: _____ ID: _____

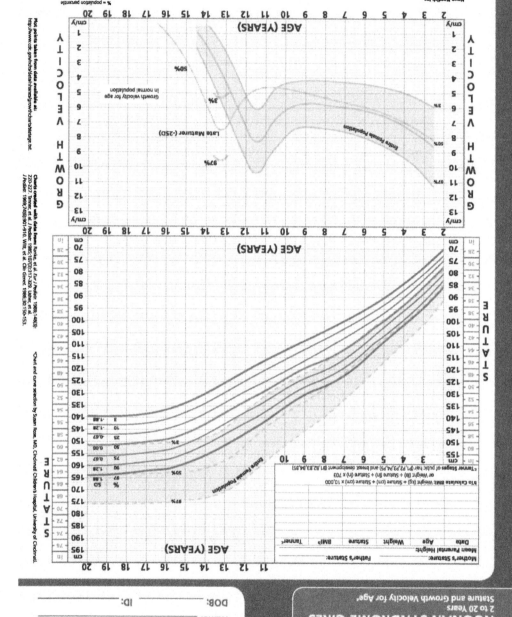

GROWTH VELOCITY

AGE (YEARS)

cm/y

Growth velocity for age
in normal population

50%

3%

97%

Late Maturer (-2SD)

Entire Female Population

STATURE

AGE (YEARS)

cm / in

3%

50%

97%

Entire Female Population

Date	Age	Weight	Stature	BMI*	Tanner*
Mother's Stature:			Father's Stature:		
Mean Parental Height:					

*Tanner Stages of pubic hair (P1,P2,P3,P4,P5) and breast development (B1,B2,B3,B4,B5)

a/b To Calculate BMI: Weight (kg) ÷ Stature (cm) ÷ Stature (cm) x 10,000
or Weight (lb) ÷ Stature (in) ÷ Stature (in) x 703

Novo Nordisk Inc.
100 College Road West
Princeton, New Jersey 08540 U.S.A.
© 2007 Novo Nordisk Inc.
132541D June 2007 Printed in the U.S.A.

% = population percentile
SD = standard deviation

Plot points taken from data available at:
http://www.cdc.gov/nchs/data/nhanes/growthcharts/chartdata/age.txt

Charts created with data from: Ranke, et al. Eur J Pediatr 1988;148(3):
220-227. Tanner, et al. J Pediatr 1985;107(3):317-329. Usher, and as in
J Pediatr 1989;74(6):901-910. Witt, et al. Clin Genet 1986;30:150-153.

*Chart and curve selection by Susan Rose, MD, Cincinnati Children's Hospital, University of Cincinnati.

novo nordisk

References 1

General papers & Guidelines

- Allanson, J. E. (1987). "Noonan syndrome." Journal of Medical Genetics 24(1): 9-13.
- Allanson, J. E. (2007). "Noonan syndrome." Am J Med Genet C Semin Med Genet 145C(3): 274-9.
- Noonan, J. A. (1994). "Noonan Syndrome: An Update and Review for the Primary Pediatrician." Clinical Pediatrics 33(9): 548-555.
- Sharland, M., M. Burch, et al. (1992). "A clinical study of Noonan syndrome." Arch Dis Child 67(2): 178-83.
- van der Burgt, I. (2007). "Noonan syndrome." Orphanet J Rare Dis 2: 4.
- Zenker, M. E. (2009). "Noonan syndrome and related disorders: A matter of deregulated RAS Signaling." Monographs in Human Genetics 17(Karger).

Anaesthesia

- Campbell, A. M. and J. D. Bousfield (1992). "Anaesthesia in a patient with Noonan's syndrome and cardiomyopathy." Anaesthesia 47(2): 131-3.
- Grange, C. S., R. Heid, et al. (1998). "Anaesthesia in a parturient with Noonan's syndrome." Can J Anaesth 45(4): 332-6.
- Lee, C. K., B. S. Chang, et al. (2001). "Spinal deformities in Noonan syndrome: a clinical review of sixty cases." J Bone Joint Surg Am 83-A(10): 1495-502.
- Macksey, L. F. and B. White (2007). "Anesthetic management in a pediatric patient with Noonan syndrome, mastocytosis, and von Willebrand disease: a case report." AANA J 75(4): 261-4.
- McBain, J., E. G. Lemire, et al. (2006). "Epidural labour analgesia in a parturient with Noonan syndrome: a case report." Can J Anaesth 53(3): 274-8.
- Ng, C. H., B. Singh, et al. (2005). "Dental anaesthesia in a patient with Noonan syndrome." Br J Oral Maxillofac Surg 43(3): 267-8.
- Sharma, P. R., U. M. MacFadyen, et al. (2007). "Dental management of a child patient with Noonan's syndrome." Dent Update 34(2): 117-8, 120.

Behaviour, Developmental Delay & Communication

- Collins, E. and G. Turner (1973). "The Noonan syndrome--a review of the clinical and genetic features of 27 cases." J Pediatr 83(6): 941-50.
- Cornish, K. M. (1996). "Verbal-performance discrepancies in a family with Noonan syndrome." Am J Med Genet 66(2): 235-6.
- Ghaziuddin, M., B. Bolyard, et al. (1994). "Autistic disorder in Noonan syndrome." J Intellect Disabil Res 38 (Pt 1): 67-72.
- Horiguchi, T. and K. Takeshita (2003). "Neuropsychological developmental change in a case with Noonan syndrome: longitudinal assessment." Brain Dev 25(4): 291-3.
- Lee, D. A., S. Portnoy, et al. (2005). "Psychological profile of children with Noonan syndrome." Dev Med Child Neurol 47(1): 35-8.
- Money, J. and M. E. Kalus, Jr. (1979). "Noonan's syndrome. IQ and specific disabilities." Am J Dis Child 133(8): 846-50.
- Money, J. and V. Duch (1981). "Adolescent males with Noonan's syndrome: behavioral and erotosexual status." J Pediatr Psychol 6(3): 265-74.
- Pierpont, E. I., M. E. Pierpont, et al. (2009). "Genotype differences in cognitive functioning in Noonan syndrome." Genes, Brain and Behavior 8(3): 275-282.
- Sarimski, K. (2000). "Developmental and behavioural phenotype in Noonan syndrome?" Genet Couns 11(4): 383-90.
- Troyer, A. K. and M. Joschko (1997). "Cognitive Characteristics Associated with Noonan Syndrome: Two Case Reportsy." Child Neuropsychology 3 (3): 199 - 205.
- van der Burgt, I. (2007). "Noonan syndrome." Orphanet J Rare Dis 2: 4.
- Verhoeven, W. M., J. L. Hendrikx, et al. (2004). "Alexithymia in Noonan syndrome." Genet Couns 15(1): 47-52.
- Verhoeven, W., E. Wingbermuhle, et al. (2008). "Noonan syndrome: psychological and psychiatric aspects." Am J Med Genet A 146A(2): 191-6.
- Wilson, M. and A. Dyson (1982). "Noonan syndrome: speech and language characteristics." J Commun Disord 15(5): 347-52.
- Wingbermuehle, E., J. Egger, et al. (2009). "Neuropsychological and Behavioral Aspects of Noonan Syndrome." Hormone Research in Paediatrics 72 (Suppl. 2): 15-23.
- Wood, A., A. Massarano, et al. (1995). "Behavioural aspects and psychiatric findings in Noonan's syndrome." Arch Dis Child 72(2): 153-5.

References 2

Bleeding

- Alanay, Y., S. Balci, et al. (2004). "Noonan syndrome and systemic lupus erythematosus: presentation in childhood." Clin Dysmorphol 13(3): 161-3.
- Bertola, D. R., J. D. Carneiro, et al. (2003). "Hematological findings in Noonan syndrome." Rev Hosp Clin Fac Med Sao Paulo 58(1): 5-8.
- de Haan, M., J. J. vd Kamp, et al. (1988). "Noonan syndrome: partial factor XI deficiency." Am J Med Genet 29(2): 277-82.
- Dineen, R. A. and R. K. Lenthall (2004). "Aneurysmal sub-arachnoid haemorrhage in patients with Noonan syndrome: a report of two cases and review of neurovascular presentations in this syndrome." Neuroradiology 46(4): 301-5.
- Emmerich, J., M. Aiach, et al. (1992). "Noonan's syndrome and coagulation-factor deficiencies." Lancet 339(8790): 431.
- Flick, J. T., A. K. Singh, et al. (1991). "Platelet dysfunction in Noonan's syndrome. A case with a platelet cyclooxygenase-like deficiency and chronic idiopathic thrombocytopenic purpura." Am J Clin Pathol 95(5): 739-42.
- Kitchens, C. S. and J. A. Alexander (1983). "Partial deficiency of coagulation factor XI as a newly recognized feature of Noonan syndrome." J Pediatr 102(2): 224-7.
- Lisbona, M. P., M. Moreno, et al. (2009). "Noonan syndrome associated with systemic lupus erythematosus." Lupus 18(3): 267-9.
- Massarano, A. A., A. Wood, et al. (1996). "Noonan syndrome: coagulation and clinical aspects." Acta Paediatr 85(10): 1181-5.
- Sgouros, S. N., G. Karamanolis, et al. (2004). "Postbiopsy intramural hematoma of the duodenum in an adult with Noonan's syndrome." J Gastroenterol Hepatol 19(10): 1217-9.
- Sharland, M., M. A. Patton, et al. (1992). "Coagulation-factor deficiencies and abnormal bleeding in Noonan's syndrome." Lancet 339(8784): 19-21.
- Sharma, P. R., U. M. MacFadyen, et al. (2007). "Dental management of a child patient with Noonan's syndrome." Dent Update 34(2): 117-8, 120.
- Singer, S. T., D. Hurst, et al. (1997). "Bleeding disorders in Noonan syndrome: three case reports and review of the literature." J Pediatr Hematol Oncol 19(2): 130-4.
- Tofil, N. M., M. K. Winkler, et al. (2005). "The use of recombinant factor VIIa in a patient with Noonan syndrome and life-threatening bleeding." Pediatr Crit Care Med 6(3): 352-4.
- Witt, D. R., B. C. McGillivray, et al. (1988). "Bleeding diathesis in Noonan syndrome: a common association." Am J Med Genet 31(2): 305-17.

Cancer & Tumours

- Addante, R. R. and G. H. Breen (1996). "Cherubism in a patient with Noonan's syndrome." J Oral Maxillofac Surg 54(2): 210-3.
- Aggarwal, A., J. Krishnan, et al. (2001). "Noonan's syndrome and seminoma of undescended testicle." South Med J 94(4): 432-4.
- Attard-Montalto, S. P., J. E. Kingston, et al. (1994). "Noonan's syndrome and acute lymphoblastic leukaemia". Med Pediatr Oncol 23(4): 391-2.
- Bader-Meunier, B., G. Tchernia, et al. (1997). "Occurrence of myeloproliferative disorder in patients with Noonan syndrome." J Pediatr 130(6): 885-9.
- Chantrain, C. F., P. Jijon, et al. (2007). "Therapy-related acute myeloid leukemia in a child with Noonan syndrome and clonal duplication of the germline PTPN11 mutation." Pediatr Blood Cancer 48(1): 101-4.
- Cheong, J. L. and M. H. Moorkamp (2007). "Respiratory failure, juvenile myelomonocytic leukemia, and neonatal Noonan syndrome." J Pediatr Hematol Oncol 29(4): 262-4.
- Choong, K., M. H. Freedman, et al. (1999). "Juvenile myelomonocytic leukemia and Noonan syndrome." J Pediatr Hematol Oncol 21(6): 523-7.
- Connor, J. M., D. A. Evans, et al. (1982). "Multiple odontogenic keratocysts in a case of the Noonan syndrome." Br J Oral Surg 20(3): 213-6.
- Cotton, J. L. and R. G. Williams (1995). "Noonan syndrome and neuroblastoma." Arch Pediatr Adolesc Med 149(11): 1280-1.
- de Lange, J., H. P. van den Akker, et al. (2007). "Central giant cell granuloma of the jaw: a review of the literature with emphasis on therapy options." Oral Surg Oral Med Oral Pathol Oral Radiol Endod 104(5): 603-15.
- de Lange, J. and H. P. van der Akker (2006). "Noonan syndrome with giant cell lesions." Int J Paediatr Dent 16(1): 69.
- Dotters, D. J., W. C. Fowler, Jr., et al. (1986). "Argon laser therapy of vulvar angiokeratoma." Obstet Gynecol 68(3 Suppl): 56S-59S.

References 3

Cancer and tumours continued...

- Edwards, P. C., J. Fox, et al. (2005). "Bilateral central giant cell granulomas of the mandible in an 8-year-old girl with Noonan syndrome (Noonan-like/multiple giant cell lesion syndrome)." Oral Surg Oral Med Oral Pathol Oral Radiol Endod 99(3): 334-40.
- Fryssira, H., G. Leventopoulos, et al. (2008). "Tumor development in three patients with Noonan syndrome." Eur J Pediatr 167(9): 1025-31.
- Fukuda, M., K. Horibe, et al. (1997). "Spontaneous remission of juvenile chronic myelomonocytic leukemia in an infant with Noonan syndrome." J Pediatr Hematol Oncol 19(2): 177-9.
- Johannes, J. M., E. R. Garcia, et al. (1995). "Noonan's syndrome in association with acute leukemia." Pediatr Hematol Oncol 12(6): 571-5.
- Jung, A., S. Bechthold, et al. (2003). "Orbital rhabdomyosarcoma in Noonan syndrome." J Pediatr Hematol Oncol 25(4): 330-2.
- Khan, S., H. McDowell, et al. (1995). "Vaginal rhabdomyosarcoma in a patient with Noonan syndrome." J Med Genet 32(9): 743-5.
- Kondoh, T., E. Ishii, et al. (2003). "Noonan syndrome with leukaemoid reaction and overproduction of catecholamines: a case report." Eur J Pediatr 162(7-8): 548-9.
- Kratz, C. P. and C. M. Niemeyer (2005). "Juvenile myelomonocytic leukemia." Hematology 10 Suppl 1: 100-3.
- Lee, S. M. and J. C. Cooper (2005). "Noonan syndrome with giant cell lesions." Int J Paediatr Dent 15(2): 140-5.
- Lee, C. K., B. S. Chang, et al. (2001). "Spinal deformities in Noonan syndrome: a clinical review of sixty cases." J Bone Joint Surg Am 83-A(10): 1495-502.
- Lopez-Miranda, B., S. J. Westra, et al. (1997). "Noonan syndrome associated with neuroblastoma: a case report." Pediatr Radiol 27(4): 324-6.
- Matsubara, K., H. Yabe, et al. (2005). "Acute myeloid leukemia in an adult Noonan syndrome patient with PTPN11 mutation." Am J Hematol 79(2): 171-2.
- Meyer, W. R. and D. J. Dotters (1996). "Laser treatment of recurrent vulvar angiokeratoma associated with Noonan syndrome." Obstet Gynecol 87 (5 Pt 2): 863-5.
- Moschovi, M., V. Touliatou, et al. (2007). "Rhabdomyosarcoma in a patient with Noonan syndrome phenotype and review of the literature." J Pediatr Hematol Oncol 29(5): 341-4.
- Mutesa, L., G. Pierquin, et al. (2008). "Germline PTPN11 missense mutation in a case of Noonan syndrome associated with mediastinal and retroperitoneal neuroblastic tumors." Cancer Genet Cytogenet 182(1): 40-2.
- Piombo, M., C. Rosanda, et al. (1993). "Acute lymphoblastic leukemia in Noonan syndrome: report of two cases." Med Pediatr Oncol 21(6): 454-5.
- Roti, G., R. La Starza, et al. (2006). "Acute lymphoblastic leukaemia in Noonan syndrome." Br J Haematol 133(4): 448-50.
- Schuettpelz, L. G., S. McDonald, et al. (2009). "Pilocytic astrocytoma in a child with Noonan syndrome." Pediatr Blood Cancer 53(6): 1147-9.
- Seeliger, T., J. U. Voigt, et al. (2004). "Pulsating thoracic tumor caused by extragenital endometriosis in a patient with Noonan syndrome." Ann Thorac Surg 77(6): 2204-6.
- Sherman, C. B., A. Ali-Nazir, et al. (2009). "Primary mixed glioneuronal tumor of the central nervous system in a patient with noonan syndrome: a case report and review of the literature." J Pediatr Hematol Oncol 31(1): 61-4.
- Sidwell, R. U., P. Rouse, et al. (2008). "Granular cell tumor of the scrotum in a child with Noonan syndrome." Pediatr Dermatol 25(3): 341-3.
- Silvio, F., L. Carlo, et al. (2002). "Transient abnormal myelopoiesis in Noonan syndrome." J Pediatr Hematol Oncol 24(9): 763-4.
- Swanson, K. D., J. M. Winter, et al. (2008). "SOS1 mutations are rare in human malignancies: implications for Noonan Syndrome patients." Genes Chromosomes Cancer 47(3): 253-9.
- Ucar, B., A. Okten, et al. (1998). "Noonan syndrome associated with central giant cell granuloma." Clin Genet 53(5): 411-4.

Cardiac

- Abadir, S., T. Edouard, et al. (2007). "Severe aortic valvar stenosis in familial Noonan syndrome with mutation of the PTPN11 gene." Cardiol Young 17(1): 95-7.
- Brown, J. R. and G. Plotnick (2008). "Pulmonary Artery Aneurysm as a Cause for Chest Pain in a Patient with Noonanâ€™s Syndrome: A Case Report." Cardiology 110(4): 249-251.

References 4

Cardiac continued...

- Burch, M., M. Sharland, et al. (1993). "Cardiologic abnormalities in Noonan syndrome: phenotypic diagnosis and echocardiographic assessment of 118 patients." J Am Coll Cardiol 22(4): 1189-92.
- Burch, T. M., F. X. McGowan, Jr., et al. (2008). "Congenital Supravalvular Aortic Stenosis and Sudden Death Associated with Anesthesia: What's the Mystery?" Anesth Analg 107(6): 1848-1854.
- Heuschmann, D., O. Butenandt, et al. (1996). "Left ventricular volume and mass in children on growth hormone therapy compared with untreated children." European Journal of Pediatrics 155(2): 77-80.
- Holt, S., Ryan, W.F., Kirkham, N., Coulshed, N. (1979). "Noonan's Syndrome and Cyanotic Congenital Heart Disease." Acta Cardiologica XXXIV(3): 167-177.
- Hudsmith, L. S. Petersen, et al. (2006). "Hypertrophic cardiomyopathy in Noonan Syndrome closely mimics familial hypertrophic cardiomyopathy due to sarcomeric mutations." The International Journal of Cardiovascular Imaging (formerly Cardiac Imaging) 22(3): 493-495.
- Kelnar, C. J. H. (2003). The role of somatropin therapy in children with Noonan syndrome. Treat Endocrinol. 2003;2(3):165-72.
- Kelnar, C. J. H. (2000). "Growth Hormone Therapy in Noonan Syndrome." Hormone Research in Paediatrics 53(Suppl. 1): 77-81.
- Kurose, A., O. Kotaro, et al. (2000). "Dilated cardiomyopathy in Noonan's Syndrome: A first autopsy case." Human pathology 31(6): 764-767.
- Leye, M., G. Calcagni, et al. (2009). "Coronary myocardial bridging in Noonan syndrome: definitive diagnosis with high-resolution CT." Br J Radiol 82(973): e8-10.
- Marino, B., M. C. Digilio, et al. (1999). "Congenital heart diseases in children with Noonan syndrome: An expanded cardiac spectrum with high prevalence of atrioventricular canal." J Pediatr 135(6): 703-6.
- Noonan, J. A. (2005). "Noonan syndrome and related disorders." Progress in Pediatric Cardiology 20(2): 177-185.
- Noordam, C., J. M. T. Draaisma, et al. (2001). "Effects of Growth Hormone Treatment on Left Ventricular Dimensions in Children with Noonan's Syndrome." Hormone Research in Paediatrics 56(3-4): 110-113.
- Ostman-Smith, I., G. Wettrell, et al. (2005). "Echocardiographic and electrocardiographic identification of those children with hypertrophic cardiomyopathy who should be considered at high-risk of dying suddenly." Cardiology in the Young 15(06): 632-642.
- Pandit, B., A. Sarkozy, et al. (2007). "Gain-of-function RAF1 mutations cause Noonan and LEOPARD syndromes with hypertrophic cardiomyopathy." Nat Genet 39(8): 1007-1012.
- Raaijmakers, R., C. Noordam, et al. (2008). "Are ECG abnormalities in Noonan syndrome characteristic for the syndrome?" European Journal of Pediatrics 167(12): 1363-1367.
- Shaw, A. C., K. Kalidas, et al. (2007). "The natural history of Noonan syndrome: a long-term follow-up study." Archives of Disease in Childhood 92 (2): 128-132.
- Silverman, B. L. and J. R. Friedlander (1997). "Is growth hormone good for the heart?" The Journal of Pediatrics 131(1, Supplement 1): S70-S74.
- Sznajer, Y., B. Keren, et al. (2007). "The Spectrum of Cardiac Anomalies in Noonan Syndrome as a Result of Mutations in the PTPN11 Gene." Pediatrics 119(6): e1325-1331.
- Yukio, I., S. Kyoko, et al. (2003). "Fibromuscular dysplasia of coronary arteries resulting in myocardial infarction associated with hypertrophic cardiomyopathy in Noonan's syndrome." Human pathology 34(3): 282-284.

References 5

Dental

- Barberia Leache, E., D. Saavedra Ontiveros, et al. (2003). "Etiopathogenic analysis of the caries on three patients with Noonan Syndrome." Med Oral 8(2): 136-42.
- Emral, M. E. and M. O. Akcam (2009). "Noonan syndrome: a case report." J Oral Sci 51(2): 301-6.
- Nelson, J. F., P. J. Tsaknis, et al. (1978). "Noonan's syndrome: report of a case with oral findings." J Oral Med 33(3): 94-6.
- Okada, M., N. Sasaki, et al. (2003). "Oral findings in Noonan syndrome: report of a case." J Oral Sci 45(2): 117-21.
- Ortega Ade, O., O. Guare Rde, et al. (2008). "Orofacial aspects in Noonan syndrome: 2 case report." J Dent Child (Chic) 75(1): 85-90.
- Sugar, A. W., A. Ezsias, et al. (1994). "Orthognathic surgery in a patient with Noonan's syndrome." J Oral Maxillofac Surg 52(4): 421-5.

Diagnosis

- Achiron, R., J. Heggesh, et al. (2000). "Noonan syndrome: a cryptic condition in early gestation." Am J Med Genet 92(3): 159-65.
- Duncan, W. J., R. S. Fowler, et al. (1981). "A comprehensive scoring system for evaluating Noonan syndrome." Am J Med Genet 10(1): 37-50.
- Ferrero, G. B. et al. (2008). "Clinical and molecular characterization of 40 patients with Noonan syndrome." Eur J Med Genet 51(6): 566-72.
- Jongmans, M., B. Otten, et al. (2004). "Genetics and variation in phenotype in Noonan syndrome." Horm Res 62 Suppl 3: 56-9.
- Jorge, A. A. L., A. C. Malaquias, et al. (2009). "Noonan Syndrome and Related Disorders: A Review of Clinical Features and Mutations in Genes of the RAS/MAPK Pathway." Hormone Research in Paediatrics 71(4): 185-193.
- Narumi, Y., Y. Aoki, et al. (2008). "Clinical manifestations in patients with SOS1 mutations range from Noonan syndrome to CFC syndrome." J Hum Genet 53(9): 834-41.
- Neri, G., J. Allanson, et al. (2008). "No reason yet to change diagnostic criteria for Noonan, Costello and cardio-facio-cutaneous syndromes." J Med Genet 45(12): 832.
- Roberts, A. E., T. Araki, et al. (2007). "Germline gain-of-function mutations in SOS1 cause Noonan syndrome." Nat Genet 39(1): 70-4.
- Sharland, M., M. Morgan, et al. (1993). "Photoanthropometric study of facial growth in Noonan syndrome." Am J Med Genet 45(4): 430-6.
- Sharland, M., M. Morgan, et al. (1993). "Genetic counselling in Noonan syndrome." Am J Med Genet 45(4): 437-40.
- Shaw, A. C., K. Kalidas, et al. (2007). "The natural history of Noonan syndrome: a long-term follow-up study." Archives of Disease in Childhood 92 (2): 128-132.
- Tramboo, N. A., K. Iqbal, et al. (2002). "Unusual dysmorphic features in five patients with Noonan's syndrome: a brief review." J Paediatr Child Health 38(5): 521-5.
- van der Burgt, I. (2007). "Noonan syndrome." Orphanet J Rare Dis 2: 4.

Gastrointestinal & Feeding

- Bitton, A., J. N. Keagle, et al. (2007). "Small bowel bezoar in a patient with Noonan syndrome: report of a case." MedGenMed 9(1): 34.
- Cumming, W. A. and J. S. Simpson (1977). "Intestinal diverticulosis in Noonan's syndrome." Br J Radiol 50(589): 64-5.
- Keberle, M., H. Mork, et al. (2000). "Computed tomography after lymphangiography in the diagnosis of intestinal lymphangiectasia with protein-losing enteropathy in Noonan's syndrome." Eur J Radiol 10(10): 1591-3.
- Sarimski, K. (2000). "Developmental and behavioural phenotype in Noonan syndrome?" Genet Couns 11(4): 383-90.
- Shah, N., M. Rodriguez, et al. (1999). "Feeding difficulties and foregut dysmotility in Noonan's syndrome." Arch Dis Child 81(1): 28-31.
- Shaw, A. C., K. Kalidas, et al. (2007). "The natural history of Noonan syndrome: a long-term follow-up study." Archives of Disease in Childhood 92 (2): 128-132.

References 6

Growth & Stature, Endocrine & Cryptorchidism

- Binder, G. (2009). "Noonan Syndrome, the RasMAPK Signalling Pathway and Short Stature." Hormone Research in Paediatrics 71(Suppl. 2): 64-70.
- Collins, E. and G. Turner (1973). "The Noonan syndrome--a review of the clinical and genetic features of 27 cases." J Pediatr 83(6): 941-50.
- Cotterill, A. M., W. J. McKenna, et al. (1996). "The short-term effects of growth hormone therapy on height velocity and cardiac ventricular wall thickness in children with Noonan's syndrome." J Clin Endocrinol Metab 81(6): 2291-7.
- Elsawi, M. M., J. P. Pryor, et al. (1994). "Genital tract function in men with Noonan syndrome." J Med Genet 31(6): 468-70.
- Kelnar, C. J. H. (2000). "Growth Hormone Therapy in Noonan Syndrome." Hormone Research in Paediatrics 53(Suppl. 1): 77-81.
- Kirk, J. M. W., P. R. Betts, et al. (2001). "Short stature in Noonan syndrome: response to growth hormone therapy." Archives of Disease in Childhood 84(5): 440-443.
- Limal, J.-M., B. Parfait, et al. (2006). "Noonan Syndrome: Relationships between Genotype, Growth, and Growth Factors." J Clin Endocrinol Metab 91(1): 300-306.
- MacFarlane, C. E., D. C. Brown, et al. (2001). "Growth hormone therapy and growth in children with Noonan's syndrome: results of 3 years' follow-up." J Clin Endocrinol Metab 86(5): 1953-6.
- Marcus, K. A., C. G. J. Sweep, et al. (2008). Impaired Sertoli cell function in males diagnosed with Noonan syndrome. J Pediatr Endocrinol Metab. Nov;21(11):1079-84.
- Nistal, M., R. Paniagua, et al. (1983). "Testicular biopsy and hormonal study in a male with Noonan's syndrome." Andrologia 15(5): 415-25.
- Nistal, M., R. Paniagua, et al. (1984). "Testicular lymphangiectasis in Noonan's syndrome." J Urol 131(4): 759-61.
- Noonan, J. A. (2006). "Noonan syndrome and related disorders: alterations in growth and puberty." Rev Endocr Metab Disord 7(4): 251-5.
- Noonan, J. A., R. Raaijmakers, et al. (2003). "Adult height in Noonan syndrome." Am J Med Genet A 123A(1): 68-71.
- Noordam, C., J. M. T. Draaisma, et al. (2001). "Effects of Growth Hormone Treatment on Left Ventricular Dimensions in Children with Noonanâ€™s Syndrome." Hormone Research in Paediatrics 56(3-4): 110-113.
- Noordam, C., I. van der Burgt, et al. (2001). "Growth hormone (GH) secretion in children with Noonan syndrome: frequently abnormal without consequences for growth or response to GH treatment." Clin Endocrinol (Oxf) 54(1): 53-9.
- Noordam, C., J. Span, et al. (2002). "Bone mineral density and body composition in Noonan's syndrome: effects of growth hormone treatment." J Pediatr Endocrinol Metab 15(1): 81-7.
- Noordam, C., P. G. Peer, et al. (2008). "Long-term GH treatment improves adult height in children with Noonan syndrome with and without mutations in protein tyrosine phosphatase, non-receptor-type 11." Eur J Endocrinol 159(3): 203-8.
- Ogawa, M., N. Moriya, et al. (2004). "Clinical evaluation of recombinant human growth hormone in Noonan syndrome." Endocr J 51(1): 61-8.
- Okuyama, A., N. Nishimoto, et al. (1981). "Gonadal findings in cryptorchid boys with Noonan's phenotype." Eur Urol 7(5): 274-7.
- Osio, D., J. Dahlgren, et al. (2005). "Improved final height with long-term growth hormone treatment in Noonan syndrome." Acta Paediatr 94(9): 1232-7.
- Padidela, R., C. Camacho-Hubner, et al. (2008). "Abnormal growth in noonan syndrome: genetic and endocrine features and optimal treatment." Horm Res 70(3): 129-36.
- Redman, J. F. (1973). "Noonan's syndrome and cryptorchidism." J Urol 109(5): 909-11.
- Romano, A. A., K. Dana, et al. (2009). "Growth Response, Near-Adult Height, and Patterns of Growth and Puberty in Patients with Noonan Syndrome Treated with Growth Hormone." J Clin Endocrinol Metab 94(7): 2338-2344.
- Sasagawa, I., T. Nakada, et al. (1994). "Gonadal function and testicular histology in Noonan's syndrome with bilateral cryptorchidism." Arch Androl 32(2): 135-40.
- Shaw, A. C., K. Kalidas, et al. (2007). "The natural history of Noonan syndrome: a long-term follow-up study." Archives of Disease in Childhood 92 (2): 128-132.

References 7

Growth & Stature, Endocrine & Cryptorchidism continued...

• Theintz, G. and M. O. Savage (1982). "Growth and pubertal development in five boys with Noonan's syndrome." Arch Dis Child **57**(1): 13-7.

• Walton-Betancourth, S., , C. E. Martinelli, et al. (2007). "Excellent growth response to growth hormone therapy in a child with PTPN11-negative Noonan syndrome and features of growth hormone resistance." J Endocrinol Invest **30**(5): 439-41.

• Witt, D. R., B. A. Keena, et al. (1986). "Growth curves for height in Noonan syndrome." Clin Genet **30**(3): 150-3.

Hearing

• Miura, M., I. Sando, et al. (2001). "Temporal bone histopathological study of Noonan syndrome." Int J Pediatr Otorhinolaryngol **60**(1): 73-82.

• Qiu, W. W., S. S. Yin, et al. (1998). "Audiologic manifestations of Noonan syndrome." Otolaryngol Head Neck Surg **118**(3 Pt 1): 319-23.

• Scheiber, C., A. Hirschfelder, et al. (2009). "Bilateral cochlear implantation in children with Noonan syndrome." Int J Pediatr Otorhinolaryngol **73**(6): 889-94.

Immune

• Alanay, Y., S. Balci, et al. (2004). "Noonan syndrome and systemic lupus erythematosus: presentation in childhood." Clin Dysmorphol **13**(3): 161-3.

• Lopez-Rangel, E., P. N. Malleson, et al. (2005). "Systemic lupus erythematosus and other autoimmune disorders in children with Noonan syndrome." Am J Med Genet A **139**(3): 239-42.

• Martin, D. M., C. F. Gencyuz, et al. (2001). "Systemic lupus erythematosus in a man with Noonan syndrome." Am J Med Genet **102**(1): 59-62.

Lymph

• Bloomfield, F. H., W. Hadden, et al. (1997). "Lymphatic dysplasia in a neonate with Noonan's syndrome." Pediatr Radiol **27**(4): 321-3.

• Cheng, M. F., Y. W. Wu, et al. (2008). "Usefulness of lymphoscintigraphy in demonstrating lymphedema in patients with Noonan syndrome." Clin Nucl Med **33**(3): 226-7.

• Evans, D. G., R. N. Lonsdale, et al. (1991). "Cutaneous lymphangioma and amegakaryocytic thrombocytopenia in Noonan syndrome." Clin Genet **39**(3): 228-32.

• Fisher, E., E. B. Weiss, et al. (1982). "Spontaneous chylothorax in Noonan's syndrome." Eur J Pediatr **138**(3): 282-4.

• Lanning, P., S. Simila, et al. (1978). "Lymphatic abnormalities in Noonan's syndrome." Pediatr Radiol **7**(2): 106-9.

• Miller, M. and A. C. Motulsky (1978). "Noonan syndrome in an adult family presenting with chronic lymphedema." Am J Med **65**(2): 379-83.

• Ogata, T., S. Sato, et al. (2003). "Lymphstasis in a boy with Noonan syndrome: implication for the development of skeletal features." Endocr J **50**(3): 319-24.

• Phillips, W. G., M. G. Dunnill, et al. (1993). "Orbital oedema: an unusual presentation of Noonan's syndrome." Br J Dermatol **129**(2): 190-2.

• Scalzetti, E. M., E. R. Heitzman, et al. (1991). "Developmental lymphatic disorders of the thorax." Radiographics **11**(6): 1069-85.

• Vallet, H. L., P. G. Holtzapple, et al. (1972). "Noonan syndrome with intestinal lymphangiectasis. A metabolic and anatomic study." J Pediatr **80**(2): 269-74.

• White, S. W. (1984). "Lymphedema in Noonan's syndrome." Int J Dermatol **23**(10): 656-7.

• Witt, D. R., H. E. Hoyme, et al. (1987). "Lymphedema in Noonan syndrome: clues to pathogenesis and prenatal diagnosis and review of the literature." Am J Med Genet **27**(4): 841-56.

Miscellaneous

• Qian, J. G. and X. J. Wang (2007). "Noonan syndrome and correction of the webbed neck." J Plast Reconstr Aesthet Surg **60**(3): 316-9.

References 8

Neurology

- Dineen, R. A. and R. K. Lenthall (2004). "Aneurysmal sub-arachnoid haemorrhage in patients with Noonan syndrome: a report of two cases and review of neurovascular presentations in this syndrome." Neuroradiology 46(4): 301-5.
- Duenas, D. A., S. Preissig, et al. (1973). "Neurologic manifestations of the Noonan syndrome." South Med J 66(2): 193-6.
- Ganesan, V. and F. J. Kirkham (1997). "Noonan syndrome and moyamoya." Pediatr Neurol 16(3): 256-8.
- Hara, T., T. Sasaki, et al. (1993). "Noonan phenotype associated with intracerebral hemorrhage and cerebral vascular anomalies: case report." Surg Neurol 39(1): 31-6.
- Heye, N. and J. W. Dunne (1995). "Noonan's syndrome with hydrocephalus, hindbrain herniation, and upper cervical intracord cyst." J Neurol Neurosurg Psychiatry 59(3): 338-9.
- Hinnant, C. A. (1995). "Noonan syndrome associated with thromboembolic brain infarcts and posterior circulation abnormalities." Am J Med Genet 56(2): 241-4.
- Holder-Espinasse M, Winter RM: Type 1 Arnold-Chiari malformation and Noonan Syndrome. A new diagnostic feature. Dysmorphol 2003;12:275.
- Kratz, C. P., G. Zampino, et al. (2009). "Craniosynostosis in patients with Noonan syndrome caused by germline KRAS mutations." Am J Med Genet A 149A(5): 1036-40.
- Rudge, P., B. G. Neville, et al. (1974). "A case of Noonan's syndrome and hypoparathyroidism presenting with epilepsy." J Neurol Neurosurg Psychiatry 37(1): 108-11.
- Saito, Y., M. Sasaki, et al. (1997). "A case of Noonan syndrome with cortical dysplasia." Pediatr Neurol 17(3): 266-9.
- Schon, F., J. Bowler, et al. (1992). "Cerebral arteriovenous malformation in Noonan's syndrome." Postgrad Med J 68(795): 37-40.
- Schuster, J. M. and T. S. Roberts (1999). "Symptomatic moyamoya disease and aortic coarctation in a patient with Noonan's syndrome: strategies for management." Pediatr Neurosurg 30(4): 206-10.
- Tanaka, Y., M. Masuno, et al. (1999). "Noonan syndrome and cavernous hemangioma of the brain." Am J Med Genet 82(3): 212-4.
- Wilms, H., B. Neubauer, et al. (2002). "Cerebral occlusive artery disease in Noonan syndrome." Cerebrovasc Dis 14(2): 133-5.
- Yamashita, Y., A. Kusaga, et al. (2004). "Noonan syndrome, moyamoya-like vascular changes, and antiphospholipid syndrome." Pediatr Neurol 31(5): 364-6.

Orthopaedic

- Butler, M. G., R. Kumar, et al. (2000). "Metacarpophalangeal pattern profile analysis in Noonan syndrome." Am J Med Genet 92(2): 128-31.
- Kobayashi, I., T. Aikawa, et al. (1986). "Noonan's syndrome with syringomyelia." Jpn J Psychiatry Neurol 40(1): 101-4.
- Lee, C. K., B. S. Chang, et al. (2001). "Spinal deformities in Noonan syndrome: a clinical review of sixty cases." J Bone Joint Surg Am 83-A(10): 1495-502.
- Mascheroni, E., M. C. Digilio, et al. (2008). "Pigmented villonodular synovitis in a patient with Noonan syndrome and SOS1 gene mutation." Am J Med Genet A 146A(22): 2966-7.
- Motohashi, O., R. Shirane, et al. (1993). "Tethered cord syndrome associated with male Turner's syndrome." Surg Neurol 40(1): 57-60.
- Naficy, S., N. T. Shepard, et al. (1997). "Multiple temporal bone anomalies associated with Noonan syndrome." Otolaryngol Head Neck Surg 116(2): 265-7.
- Sanford, R. A., R. Bowman, et al. (1999). "A 16-year-old male with Noonan's syndrome develops progressive scoliosis and deteriorating gait." Pediatr Neurosurg 30(1): 47-52.
- Sinis, N., T. I. Lanaras, et al. (2009). "Free latissimus dorsi flap with long venous grafts for closure of a soft tissue defect of the spine in a patient with Noonan's syndrome: a case report." Microsurgery 29(6): 486-9.
- Takagi, M., Y. Miyashita, et al. (2000). "Estrogen deficiency is a potential cause for osteopenia in adult male patients with Noonan's syndrome." Calcif Tissue Int 66(3): 200-3.

References 9

Prenatal

- Achiron, R., J. Heggesh, et al. (2000). "Noonan syndrome: a cryptic condition in early gestation." Am J Med Genet 92(3): 159-65.
- Bekker, M. N., A. T. Go, et al. (2007). "Persistence of nuchal edema and distended jugular lymphatic sacs in Noonan syndrome." Fetal Diagn Ther 22(4): 245-8.
- Cullimore, A. J., K. G. Smedstad, et al. (1999). "Pregnancy in women with Noonan syndrome: report of two cases." Obstet Gynecol 93(5 Pt 2): 813-6.
- Donnenfeld, A. E., M. A. Nazir, et al. (1991). "Prenatal sonographic documentation of cystic hygroma regression in Noonan syndrome." Am J Med Genet 39(4): 461-5.
- Gandhi, S. V., E. S. Howarth, et al. (2004). "Noonan syndrome presenting with transient cystic hygroma." J Obstet Gynaecol 24(2): 183-4.
- Graesslin, O., E. Derniaux, et al. (2007). "Characteristics and outcome of fetal cystic hygroma diagnosed in the first trimester." Acta Obstet Gynecol Scand 86(12): 1442-6.
- Houweling, A. C., Y. M. d. Mooij, et al. "Prenatal detection of Noonan syndrome by mutation analysis of the <I>PTPN11</I> and the <I>KRAS</I> genes." Prenatal Diagnosis 30(3): 284-286.
- Joo, J. G., A. Beke, et al. (2005). "Successful pregnancy in a Noonan syndrome patient after 3 unsuccessful pregnancies from severe fetal hydrops: a case report." J Reprod Med 50(5): 373-6.
- Kiyota, A., K. Tsukimori, et al. (2008). "Spontaneous resolution of cystic hygroma and hydrops in a fetus with Noonan's syndrome." Fetal Diagn Ther 24(4): 499-502.
- McBain, J., E. G. Lemire, et al. (2006). "Epidural labour analgesia in a parturient with Noonan syndrome: a case report." Can J Anaesth 53(3): 274-8.
- Schluter, G., M. Steckel, et al. (2005). "Prenatal DNA diagnosis of Noonan syndrome in a fetus with massive hygroma colli, pleural effusion and ascites." Prenat Diagn 25(7): 574-6.

Renal

- Barker, M. and W. Engelhardt (2001). "Bilateral kidney duplication in familial Noonan's syndrome." Clin Pediatr (Phila) 40(4): 241-2.
- George, C. D., A. Patton, et al. (1993). "Abdominal ultrasound in Noonan syndrome: a study of 44 patients." Pediatr Radiol 23(4): 316-8.
- Gupta, A., A. Khaira, et al. (2009). "Noonan syndrome: crossed fused ectopic kidneys and focal segmental glomerulosclerosis-a rare association." Clin Exp Nephrol.
- Hellebusch, A. A. (1971). "Noonan syndrome with bilateral ureteral ectopia." J Pediatr Surg 6(4): 490.
- Raghavaiah, N. V. (1975). "Noonan's syndrome associated with cake kidney." Urology 5(5): 640-2.
- Raghavaiah, N. V. (1976). "Letter: Importance of Noonan's syndrome for the urologist." J Urol 116(1): 134.
- Semizel, E., O. M. Bostan, et al. (2007). "Bilateral multiple pulmonary arteriovenous fistulas and duplicated renal collecting system in a child with Noonan's syndrome." Cardiology in the Young 17(02): 229-231.
- Tejani, A., C. Del Rosario, et al. (1976). "Noonan's syndrome associated with polycistic renal disease." J Urol 115(2): 209-11.

Skin

- Dotters, D. J., W. C. Fowler, Jr., et al. (1986). "Argon laser therapy of vulvar angiokeratoma." Obstet Gynecol 68(3 Suppl): 56S-59S.
- Fox, L. P., A. S. Geyer, et al. (2005). "Cutis verticis gyrata in a patient with Noonan syndrome." Pediatr Dermatol 22(2): 142-6.
- Hwang, S. and R. A. Schwartz (2008). "Keratosis pilaris: a common follicular hyperkeratosis." Cutis 82(3): 177-80.
- Lacombe, D., A. Taieb, et al. (1991). "Neonatal Noonan syndrome with a molluscoid cutaneous excess over the scalp." Genet Couns 2(4): 249-53.
- Lucker, G. P. and P. M. Steijlen (1994). "Widespread leucokeratosis in Noonan's syndrome." Clin Exp Dermatol 19(5): 414-7.
- Snell, J. A. and S. B. Mallory (1990). "Uterythema ophryogenes in Noonan syndrome." Pediatr Dermatol 7(1): 77-8.
- Wyre, H. W., Jr. (1978). "Cutaneous manifestations of Noonan's syndrome." Arch Dermatol 114(6): 929-30.

References 10

Vision

- Ascaso, F. J., M. A. Del Buey, et al. (1993). "Noonan's syndrome with keratoconus and optic disc coloboma." Eur J Ophthalmol 3(2): 101-3.
- Au, Y. K., W. P. Collins, et al. (1997). "Spontaneous corneal rupture in Noonan syndrome. A case report." Ophthalmic Genet 18(1): 39-41.
- Carvalho, D. R., V. V. Alves, et al. (2003). "Noonan syndrome associated with unilateral iris coloboma and congenital chylothorax in an infant." Clin Dysmorphol 12(2): 143-4.
- Dollfus, H., L. Cantenot, et al. (2001). "Bilateral iridoretinal colobomas in a child with a Noonan phenotype." Clin Dysmorphol 10(4): 299-300.
- Elgohary, M. A., P. Bradshaw, et al. (2005). "Anterior uveitis and congenital fibrosis of the extraocular muscles in a patient with Noonan syndrome." J Postgrad Med 51(4): 319-21.
- Gravholt, C. H., M. Warburg, et al. (2002). "Mild Noonan phenotype associated with coloboma of the iris and choroid." Clin Dysmorphol 11(1): 75-7.
- Hill, V., W. Griffiths, et al. (2000). "Non-bullous congenital ichthyosiform erythroderma, with ocular albinism and Noonan syndrome." Clin Exp Dermatol 25(8): 611-4.
- Kerr, N. M. and A. L. Vincent (2009). "The Novel Concurrence of Noonan Syndrome and Bilateral Duane-Like Synkinesis." J Pediatr Ophthalmol Strabismus: 1-4.
- Kleanthous, L., D. Cruz, et al. (1987). "Colobomata associated with Noonan's syndrome." Postgrad Med J 63(741): 559-61.
- Lee, N. B., L. Kelly, et al. (1992). "Ocular manifestations of Noonan syndrome." Eye (Lond) 6 (Pt 3): 328-34.
- Ram, S. P. and T. N. Krishna (1994). "Cardiopathy and ocular abnormalities in Noonan syndrome." Singapore Med J 35(4): 397-9.
- Reynolds, D. J., S. E. Rubin, et al. (2004). "Ocular manifestations of Noonan syndrome in the pediatric patient." J AAPOS 8(3): 282-3.
- Tramboo, N. A., K. Iqbal, et al. (2002). "Unusual dysmorphic features in five patients with Noonan's syndrome: a brief review." J Paediatr Child Health 38(5): 521-5.

Information for Parents

Sources of Information and Support

Support for parents and other family members is cited in the literature as being an important provision for families affected by NS. The groups listed below are useful sources of support and information.

- The Noonan Syndrome Support Group, Inc. (www.noonansyndrome.org)
  The Noonan Syndrome Support Group is an international organisation, based in the US, that aims to support families affected by NS all over the world.
  They offer information, support, and networking opportunities, and aim to improve awareness of NS and fund research into various aspects of the condition.
  They regularly broadcast webchats with medical experts in NS, and run a well-used discussion forum.
  For more information, or to join the Support Group, visit their website.

- Contact a Family (www.cafamily.org.uk)
  The Contact a Family website is for families who have a disabled child and whose who work with then or are interested to find out more about their needs. Contact A Family is the only UK charity providing support and advice to parents whatever the medical condition of their child, they have information on over 1,000 rare syndromes and can often put families in touch with each other.

- Orphanet (www.orpha.net)
  Orphanet is an online database of rare diseases and related services provided throughout Europe. It contains information on over 5,000 conditions, including Williams Syndrome, and lists specialised clinics, diagnostic tests, patient organisations, research projects, clinical trials and patient registries relating specifically to Noonan Syndrome.

- Department of Health—Personalisation (www.dh.gov.uk/en/SocialCare/Socialcarereform/Personalisation/index.htm)
  This website contains information on how the delivery of social care is being 'personalised'. This new approach uses individual budgets and direct payments to allow individuals more choice and control over the support they receive.

Acknowledgements

- The Noonan Syndrome Guideline Development Group

Expert	Institution	Review Area
Bronwyn Kerr (Condition Lead)	St Mary's Hospital, Manchester, UK	Cancer, Tumours
Ineke van der Burgt (Condition Lead)	Radboud University, Nijmegen Medical Centre, Nijmegen, the Netherlands	Diagnosis, Prenatal
Sus Biswas	Manchester Royal Eye Hospital, UK	Vision
Jill Clayton-Smith	St Mary's Hospital, Manchester, UK	Skin
Jovanna Dahlgren	Queen Silvia Children's Hospital, Gothenburg, Sweden	Cryptorchidism, Growth & Stature, Endocrine
Bruce Gelb	Mount Sinai School of Medicine, New York City, USA	Cardiac, Anaesthesia
Malgorzata Krajewska-Walasek	Instytut Pomnick-Centrum Zdrowia Dziecka, Warsaw, Poland	Behaviour, Developmental delay, Communication
Jacqueline Noonan	University of Kentucky, USA	Cardiac
Cees Noordam	Radboud University, Nijmegen Medical Centre, Nijmegen, the Netherlands	Cryptorchidism, Growth & Stature, Endocrine
Nick Plant	Royal Manchester Children's Hospital, UK	Renal
Adam Shaw	Institute of Child Health, London, UK	Hearing and Neurology
Natlin Thakker	University of Manchester, UK	Dental
Brad Williamson	Salford Royal Hospital, UK	Orthopaedic
Ellen Wingbermuhle	Vincent van Gogh Institute for Psychiatry, Venray, the Netherlands	Behaviour, Developmental delay, Communication
Rob Wynn	Royal Manchester Children's Hospital, UK	Bleeding and Immune

- The Noonan Syndrome Guideline Development Team
  Kate Strong, University of Manchester
  Pam Griffiths, University of Manchester
  Caroline Harrison, University of Manchester

- DYSCERNE: A Network of Centres of Expertise in Dysmorphology (www.dyscerne.org)

- Nowgen—A Centre for Genetics in Healthcare (www.nowgen.org.uk)

- Novo Nordisk Inc. for the use of NS growth charts

These guidelines were produced thanks to funding from DYSCERNE: A Network of Centre of Expertise for Dysmorphology (funded by the European Commission Public Health Executive Agency (DG Sanco) Project: 2006122).

Document Title: Management of Noonan Syndrome: A Clinical Guideline
Version: 1
Created: 15/2/2010
Reviewed: 00/00/0000
Review Date: 15/02/2011
Author: DYSCERNE— Noonan Syndrome Guideline Development Group
Contact details:bronwyn.kerr@cmft.nhs.uk
University of Manchester © 2010

INDEX

Note: Page numbers followed by *f* indicate figures and *t* indicate tables.

Printed in the United States
By Bookmasters